'I have no qualms referring this book to patients. The reader can explore individually not only the medical side of infertility and its management, but also the expected and unexpected emotions and feelings that may overwhelm them' Associate Professor McBride, head of general practice at the University of Notre Dame, Australia

'A practical guide that offers women support' *Australian Mother & Baby*

'It provides practical coaching tools for helping you identify and manage your emotional reactions and build resilience during this tumultuous time. It includes many questions and exercises to help clarify your thoughts and feelings, and journaling is emphasised – as is kindness and compassion to self' *Wellbeing Magazine*

'This sensitive approach provides a pathway for talking with patients about infertility' *Australian Doctor Magazine*

D1628474

Claire Hall founded her business, Authentic Empowerment, in 2004 and provides lifecoaching to individuals experiencing infertility. She has a postgraduate diploma in counselling and coaching from the Australian College of Applied Psychology. She is a Reiki master as well as a passionate advocate of people creating and succeeding in every aspect of their life.

Dr Devora Lieberman has been working in women's health for more than twenty-five years. A fertility specialist, she joined Sydney-based IVF clinic Genea in 2003. She devotes most of her clinical work to infertility and miscarriage management. Outside of her medical practice, she was a Director of the Fertility Society of Australia from 2005 to 2013, holding the office of Vice President from 2007 to 2009. Devora was a Director of Family Planning New South Wales from 2002 to 2014, and served as the organisation's President for eleven years.

EMPOWERED FERTILITY

A Practical Twelve-Step Guide

CLAIRE HALL with
DR DEVORA LIEBERMAN

Copyright © 2016 Claire Hall and Devora Lieberman

The right of Claire Hall and Devora Lieberman to be identified
as the Author of the Work has been asserted by them in accordance
with the Copyright, Designs and Patents Act 1988.

First published in 2016 in Australia and New Zealand by Hachette Australia Pty Ltd.

First published in Great Britain in 2019 by Headline Home,
an imprint of HEADLINE PUBLISHING GROUP

1

Apart from any use permitted under UK copyright law, this publication may
only be reproduced, stored, or transmitted, in any form, or by any means,
with prior permission in writing of the publishers or, in the case
of reprographic production, in accordance with the terms of licences
issued by the Copyright Licensing Agency.

Every effort has been made to fulfil requirements with regard to
reproducing copyright material. The author and publisher will be
glad to rectify any omissions at the earliest opportunity.

Cataloguing in Publication Data is available from the British Library

ISBN 9781472269737
eISBN 9781472269720

Cover design by Christabella Designs
Cover and internal images courtesy of Apolinarias/Shutterstock
Internal design by Kirby Jones and Christabella Designs

Offset in 11.04/17.29 pt Bembo Std by Jouve (UK), Milton Keynes

Printed and bound in Great Britain by Clays Ltd, Elcograf S.p.A.

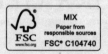

Headline's policy is to use papers that are natural, renewable and recyclable
products and made from wood grown in well-managed forests and other
controlled sources. The logging and manufacturing processes are expected
to conform to the environmental regulations of the country of origin.

HEADLINE PUBLISHING GROUP
An Hachette UK Company
Carmelite House
50 Victoria Embankment
London
EC4Y 0DZ

www.headline.co.uk
www.hachette.co.uk

Contents

Introduction

Infertility. What a loaded word. Unless you have been forced to add it to your personal vocabulary it is hard to even begin to understand its capacity to turn life upside down. But for those who have to confront it, infertility can signify a tumultuous emotional roller-coaster of pain and struggle, quietly masked behind the routines and expectations of everyday life.

Women today are able to control most aspects of their lives and make their own decisions around their personal and professional goals. And so, when faced with an infertility crisis, it often comes with an enormous shock and a feeling of your life spiralling out of control. With such a diagnosis comes feelings of anger, confusion and fear and expectations suddenly come crashing down.

Back in 2004, I was coming to the end of my studies in counselling, yet even as I received my graduate diploma,

I felt something was missing. My heart had not yet fully connected to its true purpose. Then I discovered the art of lifecoaching. Coaching is about doing things in the present to change your future, whereas counselling requires less active participation and often focuses on the past. After completing my lifecoach training, I threw off the safety wheels and pedalled as fast as I could, passionately coaching one person after another. After many years of experience, I was approached by a company to write a self-coaching program for women undergoing IVF. And so my focus turned to helping women experiencing infertility.

Through the contacts I made within that company, the name Dr Devora Lieberman was frequently mentioned. Everyone praised her professionalism and integrity and insisted I needed to meet her. So I did. It was during our first lunch that the concept of a book to assist women and their partners through IVF was born. Devora identified a gap in her patients' support process: some women simply didn't resonate with counselling and were left wading through their emotions alone. I had also been touched by the impact IVF had on several of my closest friends and often felt like a helpless bystander, unable to offer valuable assistance.

By dessert there were pages of scribbles in my notebook and the goal of a book had been set. Within days, our intention grew to reach anyone diagnosed with infertility, not just those actively experiencing IVF. It seemed the more we opened our minds to the idea of assisting women, the more we realised the need for the book.

It has only been in the past few years that I have started to develop my own approach for IVF clients, using more of a 'coachelling' model: a hybrid between coaching and counselling. When I feel a client needs further insight, I offer a deeper perspective, which is more in line with counselling than coaching. This involves a subtle shift in questions from a future focus of 'how do you want to handle this?' to a more introspective focus such as 'what happened in the past that may be affecting your thoughts?'. Once the 'aha' moment is achieved, we leap back into the action focus of coaching to bring about and hardwire the change. What this means is that this book is not one hundred per cent pure coaching – to exclude my counselling tools would feel like a disservice to you. I have kept one foot firmly planted in coaching, but occasionally dip a toe in counselling to ensure you get the best guidance possible.

It has been my privilege to coach women who have endured fertility treatment. Nothing can really prepare you for facing infertility – you cannot control its ups and downs, but you can learn to manage your reactions to it. It's not how you feel, it's how you think about how you feel at any given moment that is important. The positive results experienced by my clients fostered a need to write this book in the hope it will reach a broader audience and provide practical coaching tools to nurture self-empowerment during this taxing time. This book requires active participation to ensure the maximum results, or shifts, as I call them: a shift in perspective is all that is needed to change an experience. There are many exercises and questions throughout the book, which are designed to get you thinking differently. I suggest keeping a journal where thoughts and feelings can escape the confines of your head and begin to loosen their tight hold. It's easier to change your thinking if you can see it in black and white.

In addition to offering a coaching perspective I am privileged to have the wisdom and insight of one of Australia's leading fertility specialists, Dr Devora Lieberman. Through her vast experience she came to recognise the need for fertility coaching for many of her patients. Not only has Devora supported the development of this book, she has also referred hundreds of her patients to my office for coachelling support. Dr Lieberman weaves enormous compassion and empathy into her medical approach; she provides insight through the eyes of a fertility doctor of the emotional and physical impacts of infertility in 'The IVF Cycle Handbook' toward the end of this book.

Infertility may be holding you back from participating fully in your life, be it your relationships, career or any other area. The aim of this book is to help you uncover a path forward and women who have struggled at any point with trying to conceive will benefit from using the following steps.

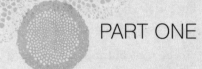

PART ONE

The Twelve-Step Guide

Before you begin

Understanding the road ahead

No two journeys are ever the same. While some women are naturally wired to take the highs and lows of infertility in their stride, many others find it traumatic and defeating. We all face things differently, so it's important not to judge, condone or ignore the way you are feeling. Not only are your thoughts important and real, they are actually your guide, and can help you understand and safely navigate this difficult road. Sometimes it is easy to identify the clues before a crisis strikes and you can then create the necessary change. At other times, life takes matters into its own hands and creates the change for you. Infertility is such a crisis and in my coaching experience, it is often the tipping point for years of emotional baggage, unaddressed and gathering dust, to suddenly come tumbling down. Infertility can make you feel like there is nowhere left to hide. But infertility is like any other of life's challenges – it calls us to attention and tells us to take action.

This guide is not about 'destination: baby' – it will not get you pregnant – but its goal is to assist you to become the person you need to be to live a full, happy and complete life – as a mother or not. Whether you are a seasoned IVF patient or just starting out on the journey, I want to equip you with the tools and resources to ride this roller-coaster and be able to step off feeling whole, connected and strong. I also want you to have a resource to share this experience with those around you – to give your partner something that will help them understand this experience from their own perspective, and also to find tools to help family and friends who want to support you but just don't know how.

So why coaching?

Coaching is about assisting an individual to create and live their best life possible. The process sets goals, follows strategies, clears out limited beliefs and uses positive psychology tools to help you create a stronger and happier version of yourself.

As a coaching topic, infertility is a challenging one. Science and human biology stand outside the laws of positive thinking, and goal setting is not enough to manifest a baby. But the focus here is about you the individual, not the goal at hand. Despite the growing research linking stress management to increased IVF success rates, my intention with this guide is not to make false and unethical promises to improve your chances. Instead, I am offering a helping hand to find the strength and resilience that is inside you, to sustain you through this experience. You may be feeling a plethora of negative emotions right now, but no matter what else is achieved, this life crisis is an opportunity to understand yourself on a deeper, more intimate level. And once this occurs, peace of mind can be found.

Gather your tools

This book is designed to help you ask questions that will unshackle you from any negative emotions you might have, such as stress, guilt, shame, regret or frustration. It will also challenge you to uncover the roots of these thoughts, which will in turn allow you to move forward more freely. The twelve steps have been framed around four key stages: the now; the roadblocks; the overcoming, and the future. No matter what point you are starting from, you can utilise the tools and exercises when you need them most.

Before we get started, though, you will need five things to help you get the most out of the journey ahead:

1. Somewhere to record your insights, like a journal (can be paper or digital)
2. Privacy
3. Time
4. The willpower to turn off all distractions, such as mobile phones
5. A commitment to be kind to and non-judgemental of yourself.

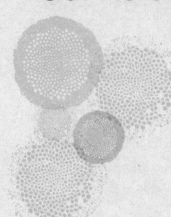

STEP 1

How Did You Get Here?

Pregnancy is supposed to be one of the most natural and rewarding experiences in a woman's life. Your mother did it, your grandmothers did it, and everyone around you may seem to be doing it too. And, of course, when you decided to get in on the action and start your own family, you never considered for a second that infertility would be a factor. But now here you are, another month gone by and still empty-handed, wondering what the heck is going on. Maybe you want to have a baby but it just hasn't happened yet and you are not sure you are ready to venture down the path of medical investigations. Maybe you are already a mother, but would love to have another child. Or maybe you have been through a few rounds of unsuccessful in vitro fertilisation (IVF) or alternative therapy and now need a new approach to build the resilience and motivation to keep trying. Whatever the reason you find yourself here, I welcome you and invite you to travel this road as a complete and satisfied person no matter what the future holds.

There may be specific reasons why you find yourself with a diagnosis of infertility, including:

1. You met your partner later in life.
2. You didn't meet a partner at all (known as social infertility).
3. Stuff happened such as caring for family or a personal crisis.
4. Work took priority.
5. You have changed your mind, having thought you didn't want children.
6. Your partner changed his or her mind and now wants children.
7. Your partner has medical issues.
8. You have medical issues.
9. You thought you had more hours left on the biological clock.

Maybe you don't even know how you got here. Whichever choices you made or were made for you cannot be changed now. Repeating them in your mind like a looping record will only cause spiralling feelings of frustration, guilt, shame, blame or anger. Recognise this as a new starting point and draw an imaginary line in the sand. Leave the past where it is, try not to concentrate too much on the future, and give your undivided attention to now, right here in this moment. Put up the white flags and call a truce with the competing parts of yourself, and focus on making peace with infertility.

This doesn't mean all the emotions of anger, blame, frustration, shame and plain old feeling sorry for yourself are not going to be with you anymore. But instead of trying to suppress the intensity of these emotions or letting them overwhelm you, try accepting that their presence is a part of your commitment on your quest to motherhood. Recognise the strength of these emotions as a sign of the importance of what you are facing, but allow them to help you validate and transform this crisis into a time of clarity, resilience and compassion.

Coaching Exercise: Your Story

Before you draw that line in the sand, you may wish to conduct a forensic investigation of how you actually got here. This is not a witch hunt for your bad decisions or the people to blame, it is about confronting your history and acknowledging it in an objective manner. The facts may be unpleasant to see but laying them all out on the table may provide new insight or perspective that is hard to uncover when everything is stuck in your head.

Ask yourself these questions to begin piecing together your fertility story:

1. What did I imagine motherhood would look like for me?

2. What derailed me from that vision?

3. What decisions were made that led me here?

4. Who, if anyone, is to blame for this?

5. What do I wish I could have done differently?

6. How do I know I made the best decisions at the time based on the knowledge I had?

As you look back at your answers, record any insights which may begin to change the way you view your story. Acknowledge the way a past decision has affected your current life; think about any benefits that decision might have brought you. You may be tempted to judge yourself for some or all of the answers, but this is the moment you must begin practising to not judge yourself.

Each time you find yourself having a negative thought about any of the answers, work through these steps. Firstly, breathe. Take five slow, deep breaths that fill up your lungs and drop your shoulders. Place your hands on your belly or one on your heart and the other on the belly; feel the air fill your belly then your chest. Exhale, feeling both areas decompress. Really connect to the simple act of breathing. This dampens the sting of the emotion. Secondly, repeat this sentence: 'I give myself permission to accept the facts as they are. It is what it is and I am ready to move on.' If there is still emotional charge, try saying, 'I am willing to forgive myself and move on'.

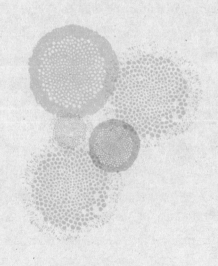

STEP 2

Accepting What Is

Accepting the naked truth is sometimes hard. An infertility diagnosis is not what you want, nor is it an accurate reflection of your efforts or prayers, but it is the truth, and as long as you are operating from this rational and factual place, you are empowered. Accepting the black and white reality is absolutely essential in moving forward on your fertility journey; don't dwell on the 'what ifs' or the 'maybes', that's mental torture. No one can say you haven't tried hard to fall pregnant. But it hasn't happened yet and sadly that is that. All you have is today, right now, and the knowledge of what today brings.

Trusting your feelings to guide you at this emotional time may not lead you to the best possible solution. Do not underestimate the trauma a diagnosis of infertility can cause to your life. Some researchers believe the stress experienced from infertility can be as great as that suffered by cancer patients, as it spreads through all areas of your life, weaving a thread of anxiety or depression. While intuition is an important tool for authentic living, when dealing with infertility, our senses can become overwhelmed and unbalanced. It's fair to say you may not be thinking clearly and intuition can unintentionally become muddled with emotional reasoning or justification. It's easy to mistake strong emotions from our lower self – the egocentric part of us – as intuitive messages from our higher self – the enlightened and loving part. Information is your key: follow your head first and then check in with your heart. If you feel you are unable to fully trust your thinking right now and are susceptible to mind tricks, then find a support person who can offer useful and objective advice and perspective. And remember, some medications, especially those used in IVF, can increase oestrogen and progesterone levels, affecting our natural thoughts and emotions. Your medical support team should help you familiarise yourself with possible side effects that may alter your perception of the world.

Just to be clear, I am certainly not suggesting entirely shutting off your emotional wisdom. How you feel is an important part of any journey, but you do not have to act upon your emotions, especially if they are compromised by hormones or stress. By keeping a journal and committing to writing a daily paragraph, you are maintaining an open dialogue with your emotions. Having an open channel to your emotions helps clear away the noise and distraction of impulsive thoughts.

I created the coaching exercise 'Learning to Accept' on page 19 to help reach your unique empowered place of acceptance and, most importantly, to stay there. From now on every thought and action needs to come from this space. It takes time and patience to gain acceptance. While working through the exercise, you may meet stubborn resistance in the form of excuses, mental blocks or a blank in your thinking. Resistance is not a bad thing; it is your subconscious keeping you safe. You may not be ready to venture down a particular path of realisation just yet and that is totally fine. Your brain is doing its job by protecting you from thoughts it can't yet process. The key is to honour and respect the resistance and give it some space and love. Try saying something to yourself like: 'I'm going to stop thinking about this now for a few days. Instead I'm going to focus on three things that make me feel comforted and loved.' This is not about denial, because in a couple of days you will return to the exercise and start the process again. Each step you take is moving you forward.

Under the surface of most acceptance issues lies fear. Fear that if we make a decision it will be the wrong one, or that we will no longer be loved, free, safe – you name it – and it's here lurking in the shadows. Fear takes on many forms, but none are insurmountable with the right guidance and faith in yourself. You really can handle anything. The sooner you accept this truth, the smoother life's challenges become.

Casey had never failed at anything in her life – she had passed every exam, excelled at netball, had climbed the career ladder in record speed. As the youngest child of five she was raised to fight for what she wanted and to never, never give up. And now she found herself confused, frustrated and irrationally angry as she embarked on her first IVF cycle. Here she was having to face her ultimate fear: the fear of failure. It was literally not an option. With all these external and internal expectations around success, Casey was unable to surrender to her infertility issues without fighting every step of the way. Through coaching, Casey began to refocus her fear of failure, and slowly came to recognise that her drive to succeed came from a wish to please. By acknowledging this pattern, Casey could then step into the realm of a strong woman who accepted uncertainty and failing as a part of her life's journey.

When you uncover a fear – the bare bones of it – it can no longer surprise you with irrational thoughts or unexpected emotions, because you know they are just expressions of its grip on your perceived vulnerability. Ever heard a strange noise in the middle of the night and been paralysed by fear? You know you have to find out what it is, but you really wish you didn't. When you finally summon up the courage to investigate, you realise it's just the wind blowing a window open, or a possum playing in the roof, and not an intruder.

You could have laid in bed for hours with heart pounding, adrenaline pumping and your ears pricked to every sound – how unnecessary and totally exhausting. Instead, by facing your fear head on, it no longer exists. The power of the unknown is gone.

Coaching Exercise: Learning to Accept

Before you start this next exercise, take a moment to recall anything you have had to accept in the past, such as your parents' divorce, not becoming a ballerina, or your crooked nose. Do you remember how you began to accept things for what they were? Was it easy or hard? Did it bring up new challenges or surprises? How long did it take? What strengths or vulnerabilities did you learn about yourself? Always jot down any insights for later reading. I want you to use this exercise for any thoughts and feelings you are struggling with at the moment. Write down at least ten pressing thoughts and feelings. For example, 'Month after month I keep failing,' 'I just want one more baby,' 'I am so selfish and ungrateful,' 'I am so ashamed,' 'I blame myself for starting late,' 'My body has failed me,' 'I am so alone,' 'It's all my fault,' 'It's all his fault,' 'My mother is so insensitive,' 'This is what I deserve for being indecisive for so long,' or 'I only want to be a mother'.

Read through each of your statements and ask yourself:

1. Does this thought take me toward empowerment?
2. Is it even true?

3. Does this thinking bring compassion and kindness to me or others?

If you answer 'no' to any of these questions, then let the thought go and clear it out. Give yourself permission to simply stop thinking about it. If it creeps back into your thinking, just say to yourself, 'I have let this go,' and clear it out again.

If you answer 'yes' to any of these questions, what do you need to do about it? If there is something you need to change, such as protecting yourself from the insensitive comments of your mother, plan and action how you will do this. If you find yourself resisting, concentrate on a positive sentence such as 'I can handle this' or 'this is only one step of many I am willing to take'.

Please don't judge your words, just witness them and imagine your best friend explaining this to you. How you would respond? With love and compassion, of course. So why should you treat yourself differently?

When you complete the exercise, be mindful of clues hidden in your writing that allow you to uncover how you speak to yourself, what thoughts aren't really your own, or which possibly reveal an empowering self-belief you had tucked away. Hopefully at the end of the exercise, the energy behind some of the things you are struggling to accept will start to move. By bringing thoughts out of the dark, you are able to perform a scathing reality check on anything that sabotages you and put it in the bin.

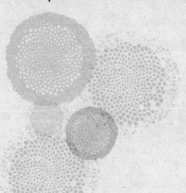

STEP 3

Letting Go of
Expectations

The thing to do to understand yourself on a deeper, more intimate level and help find greater inner peace is to examine your expectations. An expectation is a strong belief that something will happen in the future. As a human being, you are constantly generating internal and external dialogues stating what you expect to happen in life. Setting expectations helps you make sense of what is going on around you, and provides you with a sense of stability by creating a reference framework; you seek comfort from this supposed knowing. You can expect the best or you can expect the worst in life – either way, you are subjecting your mind's energy to a future reality that doesn't technically exist. So it's clear to say your expectations are not real, they are your perceived reality of how you envision your future.

Creating expectations helps minimise feelings of discomfort or stress brought about by life's uncertainty.

Your brain likes predictability and when you have your expectations met, it sends out a chemical called dopamine, which makes you feel good. The state of feeling good can become addictive, so you strive to meet more and more of your expectations to reach that same high. This can become a continuous cycle of trying to feel good or, in other words, a cycle of wanting to avoid pain. As you strive for your next dopamine hit, you may distance yourself from the expectation that sometimes things do go wrong. You can even begin to believe it is not acceptable to experience pain in the form of disappointment, frustration or other uncomfortable emotions. You want to avoid the discomfort of things going wrong, and may begin to label these experiences as bad, terrible or, even worse, not normal.

Infertility breaks this feel-good cycle because circumstances are outside your control. Instead of a dopamine hit, the stress hormone cortisol gets released into your system from the fight-or-flight area of your brain and cortisol can have negative effects on your body as well as your mind.

Managing expectations

It is very easy to label your infertility experience as really bad, terrible, unfair or dreadful – of course it is. But using such language reduces your ability to think clearly and approach the problem from the most sophisticated part of your brain, where solutions are created. This area is called the prefrontal cortex. By using this part of your brain and labelling your experiences with balanced, neutral or even positive language, it is possible to better manage your expectations. For example, instead of using the words 'hopeless' or 'heartbreaking' to describe your diagnosis, try labelling it 'a sad fact of life' or 'something that we just have to get through'. I shall go into this in more detail in Step 6: Releasing Control on page 61.

Sometimes your expectations are driven by a need to feel validated, accepted or simply normal. It's only natural to want to fit in and belong. Rarely do you consciously choose your expectations. Early childhood relationships with parents, teachers, siblings, friends and others are your earliest influencers and plant the need to expect things a certain way. According to research, the human brain is not fully mature until approximately twenty-five years of age. Until then, external influences play a large role in the programming of beliefs. Once you reach your mid-twenties, you are less dependent on certain people for your emotional and physical wellbeing, and your expectations around beliefs and habits can be suitably challenged – you have your own experiences to draw upon and are less likely to struggle to challenge the status quo from fear of rejection. Nevertheless, these early influencers are hard to shake, and it's totally natural to follow your thoughts and expectations instinctively rather than question why you think the way you do.

It can be very hard to unwire an expectation in your mind. It has been your guiding compass and served you, either positively or negatively, for a very long time. Not being able to meet your expectations, despite having all the will in the world, can be disappointing, terrifying and sometimes confidence-destroying. You might take it to mean you have failed or you aren't good enough to get what you want or, most harmfully, you are not worthy. Of course none of these statements are true, it is just your interpretation of reality – a story you tell yourself so it all makes sense. Understandably, it is easier to believe your story than sit in the agonising territory of the unanswerable 'Why?'

Before Jessica began infertility treatment, she read a statistic that said ninety per cent of pregnancies will happen within the first three attempts. This expectation had set in her mind, so after three unsuccessful rounds of IVF, Jessica believed she was never going to get pregnant. This unfulfilled expectation sent her spinning into a state of despair. Unable to think clearly for herself, she asked her doctor if this statistic was true.

The doctor told Jessica that her demographic group and individual circumstances meant success was more likely after six attempts rather than three, but cautioned her about relying too heavily on such figures.

This new information rewired Jessica's expectations of IVF and dampened her raw emotions. After discussing its impact during a coaching session, she later decided to drop the statistic altogether as this new expectation of six cycles added additional pressure in the long term. By rewiring her expectations, she chose to concentrate on putting her energy into the belief that IVF is a long-term process that she could fully commit to and therefore failed attempts were just part of the process.

Detaching from expectations

It is attachment to expectations that can cause the most harm. Attachment is an invested emotional and physical energy in the desired result; when you are not attached to something, you are able to flow with life and adapt to circumstances quicker to find the best solution, fast. Flexibility and adaptability are two key foundations that must be fostered in order to maintain a balanced approach to life. Your expectations need to resemble waves that ebb and flow according to what serves you at the time. For example, you can choose to expect to fall pregnant naturally because that's the way it should be, or you can choose to accept there is some need for additional assistance and seek medical advice sooner rather than later. The quicker you explore your thinking and uncover your driving expectations, challenge their validity and reframe them with flexibility and adaptability, the quicker you will find a practical solution.

Remember, life isn't fair and you are not the same as everyone else. You are you, with your unique partner, your unique body and your unique journey. We all wish to be excluded from the heartache of infertility, but we are only human. Bad things happen to good people and good things happen to bad people. This is not the time to challenge your deity on the unfairness of life, it's the time to clear out any sabotaging expectations and replace them with kind, supporting ones. The journal exercise on the following page can help you achieve this.

When you let go of any rigid expectations of pregnancy, you unshackle yourself from the mental torture of not living up to them. You free yourself from a self-imprisoned 'should' reality and open yourself up to the opportunities that lie ahead. You are not the first woman to experience fertility issues and you won't be the last. You are not alone, although your journey is unique to you. Start to allow yourself permission to let go and change the narrative of your story around fertility.

> Peta had spent three years believing pregnancy would just naturally happen. The first year she had idly gone about her business with her partner, Jack, with the expectation that it takes at least a year to fall pregnant. Nothing happened. By the second year, Peta had started to see her friends falling pregnant within a few months of

trying. She started to question her initial expectation and although she remained patient, panic started to set in. By the end of year two, Peta was in a whirl of pregnancy tests, alternative therapies and supplements. Determined to make the next year 'the year of falling pregnant', Peta began to feel extreme stress and pressure to live up to her expectation of falling pregnant naturally. There had been little discussion of medical intervention despite Jack bravely broaching the subject, because Peta would not accept there was possibly a problem. It was only when Peta found herself slumped over the bathroom sink in floods of tears, with a desperate Jack pleading with her to see a doctor, that she finally surrendered her need to control the situation. Peta had to accept life was not matching her expectations and that the stress she was putting on herself was causing more harm than good.

Journal Exercise

Keeping a journal is a great way to release your thoughts and emotions as well as document what is going on for you at this moment in time. In your journal, list your expectations of a future pregnancy, and be honest with yourself.

Ask yourself the following questions:

- What are my expectations around falling pregnant?
- Where did they come from originally?
- Are they flexible or rigid?

- How do they currently serve me?
- What exactly do I think when it comes to falling pregnant?
- What do I believe my partner thinks? Parents? Friends?
- What influences do I have around me that affect my viewpoint?

Try to write ten expectations. Now look at the words you use. Are they rigid, negative or vague generalisations, such as 'I should be able to fall pregnant easily just like everyone else'? Or do they suggest flexibility and adaptability to move with your circumstances, such as 'I accept there are many ways to have a baby'?

It is easier to change the nature of your expectations if your brain has evidence to support fluid and open thinking. Consider other areas of your life where you thought something would happen one way but it ended up happening totally differently. Having an open and fluid mind takes practice; your ability to surrender to the knowledge that expectations are a product of your brain mechanics rather than enlightened wisdom means you can observe these thoughts and give them less importance. Your focus must lie on what is possible outside the realms of your current thought patterns.

Coaching Exercise: Cultivate Gratitude

You don't have to look far to find scientific, religious or spiritual literature to support the power of gratitude. Gratitude is the ability to give thanks and is an act of appreciation, and cultivating an attitude of gratitude can help you manage the negative effects of expectations. You may feel you have very little to be grateful for right now, but try to push past those emotions to widen your perspective and challenge your brain to seek out what is working from what isn't. Over time, this actually rewires your brain to automatically seek out the positive in life and become naturally more solution focused.

Set aside five to ten minutes a day to reflect on three things you can be grateful for each day. You can either say these out loud or write them in your journal. Perhaps you savour your first coffee of the day or notice how fit and able your elderly parents are. By focusing on these things, you are broadening your awareness outside of your current fertility issues and staying connected to life in a positive way. It may sound silly, but try it for two disciplined weeks and feel the results. Why not ask your partner to join you?

Use these words to get started:

Today I am grateful for …

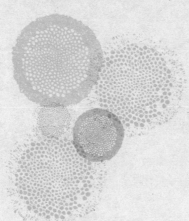

STEP 4

Feeling a Bit Off-Kilter?

You could be forgiven for thinking something has come loose upstairs in the mechanics of your brain. Your emotional state could start to resemble someone in an Alfred Hitchcock movie – unpredictable, extreme and slightly unhinged. Do not underestimate the impact of stress. The human brain acts differently when confronting a crisis. Instead of sending energy to the executive part of your brain, the prefrontal cortex (that sophisticated part I mentioned earlier), energy is diverted to the fight-or-flight area of the brain called the amygdala. It's hard to think straight when this area of the brain gets activated, since it's the primitive survival instincts centre. I think of it as the panic room.

It is believed that our basic human need, beyond anything else, is for social contact. This need even surpasses our general need for food and water, because without another human being to provide the milk to you as a baby, you wouldn't survive. Our brains are naturally wired to be social and inclined to want to stay in tribes – we rely on others to nurture and protect us. There is a perceived safety in numbers that improves our chance of survival. If we feel we don't belong to a tribe, such as our work colleagues or family and friends, then our brains perceive this isolation as unsafe or threatening. The brain is wired to detect and eradicate sources of threat and danger as quickly as possible. This goes back to early human times when our survival depended on it. Obviously, our physical danger is not on such high alert as it was in prehistoric times, but our brains are still continually scanning for potential threats.

Interestingly, our brain registers non-physical or social threats in the same area as it does physical danger – it does not clearly distinguish between the two. Therefore, you need to acknowledge the impact of social pain as you would any physical pain, because it can hurt just as much. Infertility can make you feel like an outsider and it can be tough to talk about even with close family and friends, for fear of how they may react. Remember the old saying, 'Sticks and stones may break my bones but words will never hurt me'? If you were ever teased at school you will recall this isn't exactly true: what people say can and often does affect you deeply. And because infertility is often a private and personal affair, choosing people to share your struggles with can be a fraught process, because there are rarely any physical signs of trauma, yet the emotional pain can be unbearable.

Dealing with an amygdala hijack

In order to begin to calm down the amygdala (the panic room) to release energy and focus back into the prefrontal cortex (sophisticated thinking), you need to be aware what triggers the amygdala and hijacks your emotions. Firstly, the amygdala is highly effective at keeping you safe and you need to acknowledge this. You will never be able to turn off the amygdala, but by consciously monitoring your thoughts and feelings you become better skilled at detecting the unconscious triggers and threats, and managing their effects. Eventually you will move from unconscious negative reacting to conscious positive responding – kind of like turning off the autopilot and settling into the driver's seat of your life.

Neuroscientists have discovered that one of the biggest social triggers to the amygdala is status. The brain is constantly scanning the pecking order in any social situation to determine where you stand in relation to everyone else. It's a basic survival mechanism. If you find yourself doing or saying something that goes down well with other people, then the brain releases dopamine as a reward and it basically makes you feel good. You learn to want more of that good feeling, so you try to raise your status more. For example, if you make a joke at a party and everyone laughs, you feel good about yourself. However, if your joke crashed and burned you would be left with a release of cortisol, the stress hormone, rushing through your veins as your brain sends the message there is now a social threat of rejection, and there might be a fight-or-flight situation ahead.

In fertility terms, the longer it takes to fall pregnant, the more your own feelings of self-worth within a group can be challenged, making you more susceptible to negative emotions generated by listening to others announce their due dates, attending baby showers and potentially being questioned about when you are going to start a family. When friends and colleagues become pregnant, your brain reacts to the situation as a type of threat – your failure to become pregnant indicates a lowering of your status within the group. You become hypersensitive to the situation, leading to the release of cortisol. You may find yourself feeling resentful, angry or jealous at others' joyful news simply because the mechanics of your brains are programmed to do so. Worse still is feeling guilty about these emotions. Take comfort in the fact it's not you, it's your instinctive danger mechanism setting in – every time you hear of a new pregnancy and your brain fires off feelings such as anger, jealousy and guilt, it comes from a sense of fear.

By recognising these negative emotions as part of your brain's natural reaction, and not part of your higher self, you can lessen the burden of sadness and shame they create. They are a human emotional process that you need to move through. By acknowledging emotions for what they are ('I'm feeling resentful that Jane is pregnant'), you can counter their intensity and move through them faster. Denying them can lead to the old saying 'what you resist persists', so it's best to confront the emotion head-on. Recognise that it does not mean you are less of a person if you react negatively to other women's pregnancies or motherhood journeys, and get back to focusing on what is working well in your life at this moment in time.

We need to belong

Another neuroscience discovery is that the brain likes social connection. In addition to needing a social group for mere survival, humans seek each other out for a sense of belonging. This is particularly challenging when you aren't a member of the 'pregnancy club'. A client of mine experienced four pregnancy announcements in the space of one week and her brain was emotionally hijacked by the social exclusion, which translated the threat into intense feelings of isolation and a yearning to belong. She felt victimised and became withdrawn. Again, the truth is not that she was being victimised or excluded from the pack, she was just on a different journey to them.

To find the strength to deal with such situations and still feel connected with the people around you, you need to find new terms. It is acceptable to place new boundaries around yourself and these boundaries may involve protecting your feelings and being kind to yourself. One way to keep connected is through common interests such as an evening course or spending time at a gallery discussing a new exhibition. Discovering new areas for conversation helps keep the focus off the personal.

Couples may also feel the need to exclude their tribe from their private heartache. While it is reasonable to keep secrets from friends and family, you must remember they are unaware of your distress and are not responsible for unintentionally making you feel excluded or disconnected. After all, would they intentionally want to hurt you? Of course not.

Resolve to make peace with the fact you are having a difficult time, which you may not wish to share publicly. And this is totally fine as long as you know you still belong to your social circles and in time you will find a better way to connect with the people you love.

Lay out your options

Another key factor that triggers the amygdala is lack of options. The brain loves choice and when your options are taken away or narrowed, it can automatically set off a warning that a threat is imminent. Infertility is an obvious catalyst for raising a red flag around lack of choice. The injustice and unfairness that natural conception is either not working or has been taken from you is hard for most women to process, especially since options for coping with infertility – from alternative therapies or medical interventions to fostering and adoption – are limited.

To help reduce the chance of an amygdala hijack on your emotions, look at how many options you have, not how many you don't have. Being aware of how a perceived lack of options can trigger an emotional response is a great tool to help reprogramme your mind away from fear. Of course it may feel like you have limited options to move forward, but hopefully the reality is slightly different. I once met a very elderly gentleman on a long-haul flight. We only spoke for about twenty minutes but in that short time he told me about his late wife and how they had lost six pregnancies and never had children. They would have been trying in the 1950s, which meant there was very limited medical knowledge to assist them on their agonising journey. Today there are a host of options. When you begin to notice thoughts or feelings around lack of options, remember that you are living in an age when IVF is a miracle in itself, not to mention all the alternative therapies that we now have. Practise focusing on what is available, to combat any strong emotions telling you otherwise.

Assessing fairness

Have you ever noticed how movies play on our human obsession with equality? No one wants the baddie who steals, cheats and does other nasty things to win because that's not fair. Fairness or equality is something intrinsic to our nature. The brain wants to be given rights and to be treated fairly. It loves win–win situations and gets triggered when things aren't so. Imagine your fury if you found out your work colleague was getting a huge pay rise and you weren't! Sadly, there is nothing fair about experiencing infertility. You may feel outraged at the injustice of it all and that's okay – it's not fair and it's not what you deserve. No one deserves to experience the physical and emotional challenges of infertility, but this is life and life isn't fair.

Don't let your anger build out of control – shift the energy by bashing a pillow, smashing some plates or going for a long run. You are entitled to feel the unfairness, but remember it is exacerbated by your brain's mechanics – the situation is unfair but it's not final. Hopefully, you are reading this with the knowledge that there are still options available to you for starting a family. Letting go of the expectation that life is fair is an important step in coming to terms with the fact you may not have the same journey to parenthood as most of your friends. When you can begin to accept that this is okay, you will be less triggered by the brain's desire for fairness.

Coaching Exercise: Clearing out Your Limiting Beliefs

If you are feeling brave, then why not tackle a limiting belief? I often find clients are also struggling with a career, relationship or personal dilemma in addition to their fertility issues. This is a great exercise to clear out old and out-of-date beliefs and test drive a new and improved way of thinking for confidence and motivation outside your fertility issues.

Start a list of your old limiting beliefs around the area in your life where you want to create change. For example, 'I hate working for that company', or 'I know my husband thinks I nag him'. You may want to do this exercise over a few days as you become more aware of the thoughts rolling around inside your head.

Opposite each limiting belief, write down a new empowering belief. Watch your language, and make sure you focus on the positive …

Old belief	New belief
• I have to stick with this job even though I hate it	• I am open to exploring new job possibilities
• I am scared of failing and not being good enough at work	• I am intelligent and got my job because I am capable
• Everyone's needs are more important than mine.	• I am allowed to meet my own needs and can still help others.

Now pick one or two beliefs that, if you were to integrate them into your being, would create significant positive change. Answer the following questions to gain greater clarity and confidence:

What are the old and new beliefs I want to work on?

What will I have to give up if I change this belief?

What will I allow into my life with this new belief?

What excuses crop up when I start to make the change?

What am I going to do about it?

Integrate these new beliefs into your daily life, for example, as an affirmation or by writing them on a piece of paper that you can display somewhere where it will be seen every day.

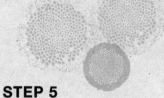

A Conversation with Fear

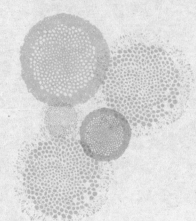

Infertility can stir feelings of fear even in the most optimistic and courageous of women. Fears such as never having a baby, fear of actually being pregnant, fear of miscarriage, fear of failure, fear of needles, to name but a few. As mentioned earlier, fear is not something we human beings naturally handle well. Fear is normally a symptom of an underlying belief that you are not safe or in control. Fear can often be a lack of knowledge, a stretch out of a comfort zone or challenging circumstance, which requires a new level of thinking. Fortunately, you can learn to live with fear and change the narrative behind its power in order to function effectively in your day-to-day life. Throughout my years of coaching there has always been one key theme when it comes to addressing fear: not taking action. Ignoring a fear can be a catalyst for anxiety and magnifies the fear. It is important to keep moving, no matter if it's a tiny step or a giant leap.

Gathering information is one of the best ways to alleviate the risk of letting your fear create an emotional hijack. Hours spent on the internet researching theories, therapies and forums is a powerful ally when addressing a knowledge gap. However, arming yourself with information should come with a warning. Remember that your brain is not designed to differentiate between a healthy behaviour and an unhealthy one – it just wants to minimise the initial risk by seeking the quickest path to alleviate the discomfort of fear. But countless hours sitting in front of the computer or in bed with your iPad can sometimes become an addictive habit that moves from an empowering informative process to an obsessive need for control. And we all know the unlimited potential of Google when we are determined to find an answer. There is a fine line between meeting a need and wanting to fulfil an insatiable desire. It's easy to slip into repeatedly searching the internet but finding little pleasure or constructive use from it. If you find yourself scanning informative resources more out of habit than need, it's time to stop and rethink.

Set yourself up for success not failure, get clear on what you need to know, what internet or information source you are going to trust and how long you are going to dedicate each day or week to researching. I suggest you cap your research time to fifteen minutes a day if you feel it is getting out of hand. And please do not read anything that is going to intensify your fear or exaggerate it. That does not serve anyone, least of all you. Keep things in perspective as much as you can. There is no miracle answer waiting for you online. It's unlikely reading 'just one more' forum is going to change everything. Your journey is completely unique to you and by surrounding yourself with the best professionals you can find, you are doing everything humanly possible. Try to find strength and comfort in that.

People are passionate about their successful fertility stories and want to inspire others by sharing their journey. You may find yourself comforted or even inspired by what you read. It is good to surround yourself with hope and positivity, as they help to shift your focus to what does work rather than what doesn't. However, by seeking an external source of comfort you are leaving yourself vulnerable to that critical voice inside your mind that can easily cast a dark shadow over your optimism. You know the one: she sounds something like, 'That's all very well for them but not all of us are that lucky', or 'Don't get your hopes up, girlfriend.'

As unlikely as it sounds, you do not have to read endless stories to achieve that sense of comfort and reassurance – you can attain it from within. By connecting to the deep sense of self, your higher self where your mind's loving wisdom can be heard over the daily noise of inner chatter, you open up a telephone line to all the good you have inside you. Meditation, yoga, relaxation or visualisation are some steps you can take to quieten the inner critic and tap back into your all-loving and powerful self. Whenever you are feeling fearful, access what your higher self believes to be true and let it override the lower self's need for fearful negative thinking. It feels like swimming in a freshwater lake after wading through thick mud. For example, an hour of yoga, meditation or massage may be enough to quieten the inner dialogue. Once relaxed, spend ten minutes writing or speaking to your higher self. Ask her direct questions and wait patiently for the response.

Ruby had experienced three unsuccessful rounds of IVF and two miscarriages. Having a baby was as important to her as breathing. She became obsessed with finding her fertility answers online despite employing the best doctor and Chinese herbalist she could find. Both had bombarded her with new information after each miscarriage and the only way she could begin to cope was to understand exactly what each was telling her – and that involved many late nights spent in online forums.

At first Ruby found great comfort and support by reading and sharing her journey. She relayed information back to her partner, Lucy, and together they discussed the merits and flaws. But Ruby gradually came to spend more and more time reading and scouring the web for information, but without experiencing any comfort and control. She found it harder and harder to hold a normal conversation with friends, let alone spend quality time with Lucy. She would start her day by logging onto forums during breakfast, read medical reports on the bus, snatched minutes at work to find new websites and ended her day in bed with the iPad glowing in the dark. Her mind was constantly distracted and her life outside of her fertility treatments was suffering.

Luckily Ruby was able to rein in her habit and recognise this destructive pattern before it cost her. She put a timetable together that allowed her to read fertility-related topics before mentally and physically pushing the topic to the side during the rest of the day. She took up meditation and breathing exercises to help her relax when the feelings became overpowering.

The power of words

Mind your Ps and Qs means 'mind your manners', 'mind your language', 'be on your best behaviour'. This is a powerful and appropriate statement that will serve you well. The words you speak are a direct indication of the way you think. The way you speak, either internally or externally, reflects and dictates the way you feel and see yourself in the world. Basically, if you see the glass as half full, then the world will be perceived through a half-full lens. This creates a positive, optimistic and solutions–focused way of living. But if you see the glass as half empty, life can seem hard, a struggle and as if you are swimming upstream. I recently asked my 93-year-old grandfather the secret to his longevity. He replied, 'It's no secret, I just expect the best to happen and it normally does.' Your thoughts really do create how you experience your reality.

I am not, however, suggesting an unrealistic 'Pollyanna' take on life, I'm merely encouraging you to carefully choose the words you use. Remember, words can have a powerful impact on your brain and the way you see yourself in the world. For example, if you find yourself saying, 'It's all hopeless and I am such a big fat failure,' then you might as well pick up the nearest stick and beat yourself. Such a statement only fuels feelings of hurt, shame, sadness and anger, and makes it impossible to act from a positive and motivating place. And if your actions are not in alignment with finding the best fertility solution, then you are not putting yourself in the greatest position to successfully address your problems. Of course you are allowed to feel these emotions – they are normal, natural and human. And getting them out either verbally or physically is crucial to keep your energy moving. But exacerbating them from a limiting and undisciplined mindset is unnecessary and pointless.

Be extremely careful how you speak to yourself and the outside world – use neutral statements if positive ones are too much of a stretch. Try to take the emotional firecracker out of a statement to defuse its negative impact on your mind and body. State the reality, not your interpretation of the facts. It's easy to get swept up in the emotional whirlwind, but this won't serve you well in the long term.

Try replacing 'but' with 'and' in your sentences as this can bring two competing realities together to find a solution. For example, 'I really want to lose ten kilos but I find it too hard to stick to a diet,' compared to, 'I really want to lose ten kilos and I find it hard to stick to a diet, so I'd better find a better way that works for me.'

Leaving a successful legacy

A common fear I often hear is around legacy. 'What is my legacy if I don't have children?' 'Why am I on the planet if it's not to have children and leave my mark as a parent?' 'Will I be alone if I don't have a family?' 'Who will be there for me when I am old?' 'What about all this love I have to give?' 'Why am I judgemental of others with children?' 'Why am I holding myself back from the children already in my life?' 'Do I believe I only have enough love for my own children?'

These are not questions for the faint-hearted. Some women will go through their entire life and never have to face such heart-wrenching honesty. It's not easy facing your fears, but it is a heck of a lot harder to keep running away from them. Again, here is an opportunity to learn more about yourself, how you think, what you want your life to stand for and to unshackle yourself from inauthentic values or needs.

So, how can you manage your beliefs around your legacy? Is being alone your greatest fear about not having a family? Are you allowing yourself to imagine future scenarios that may never exist? When people say they want to be successful, they rarely know what success would actually look like – instead they use other people's ideals to create their own. When you think about having a family, and creating a legacy, where do your thoughts come from? Have you been brought up with the expectation of having a family? How powerful were the female influences in your upbringing? What are your family's cultural values? Do you feel pressured to produce grandchildren? Has anyone in your family led a happy life without children? Do you know women who have led inspirational lives yet not had children of their own? Think of Oprah Winfrey, Kylie Minogue or Mother Teresa. Do you know of any other way you can create a powerful legacy on the planet, regardless of raising children or not? What if your actions today were an inspirational legacy in itself?

By feeling the acute pain of not leaving a legacy behind every time you are reminded of your infertility, you will struggle to properly function at work, home or life in general. And by forming a victim mentality, a 'woe is me' outlook on life, it's easy to channel your pain into anger – which is a more manageable emotion to handle in the world than raw vulnerability and pain. Because such a coping strategy has no healthy competition, anger soon gets hardwired into your brain and its many masks take hold in every aspect of your life. If you do find yourself regretting events in the past, revisiting emotive memories or daydreaming about countless 'what ifs', remember that it's okay and totally natural. You are on a very painful journey. Give yourself a break. Set a timer for ten minutes where you can let it all out and feel the raw pain of the emotions. Once the alarm beeps, stop, and get back to business.

Sally had nine failed IVF cycles and was becoming very skilled at proving that life treated her badly. She found herself being able to demonstrate she was a victim in all areas of her life. It was becoming a self-fulfilling prophecy, with bad things constantly happening. Her mother had cut off communication, she didn't get the job promotion she wanted and her house was flooded by a vindictive washing machine – the list just kept growing. Sally could justify exactly why she was a victim simply by reaffirming her belief that life had to be hard. She could never accept advice or help from someone else to solve a problem as this would go against that subconscious belief that 'life is hard' – instead she would waste energy reinventing the wheel just to prove her point.

With coaching, Sally was catapulted into a new way of thinking. Something in her brain was craving change and she immediately identified all the ways her inner critic, her 'crazy monkey' as she called it, was running wild. We could have spent hours discussing the latest evidence or drama that fuelled her philosophy, but I decided we needed to get down to the core of these victim symptoms. Sally was scared of not leaving a legacy, a piece of herself, on the planet after she died. She believed that we are all meant to leave something behind through our children and what was to come of her if she couldn't have a child?

Sally began to realise she was holding back from the beautiful children she already had in her life. This was not something she had done consciously, but deep down, the act of not giving wholly was fuelling the victim mindset and keeping her further from her truth. Sally had a wealth of love to give, which she thought she had to keep stored up for her own future family. When she made the decision to start giving that love to the children around her, she was able to unshackle herself from the self-imposed chains that kept her tied to the future. This in turn created a legacy, which was so important to her. Sally decided to no longer fuel her unconscious need to protect herself from the emptiness of not having her own children, but instead to channel the pain into an abundance of love and joy. Sally no longer had space to be a victim when life was rich with beauty, and her heart felt lighter.

Once you know better, you do better

It is important to not judge, criticise or chastise yourself when you learn something new about your ways of behaviour. I follow the belief 'once you know better, you do better'. When you are unaware of the mechanics of your brain's responses to stressful events, you cannot be held responsible for the habits that form. Your brain wants to minimise potential threats and keep you as safe as possible, both physically and emotionally. The truth is your brain will always serve you the best way it can. Unfortunately, though, it doesn't know how to distinguish between a healthy habit or a sabotaging one – its only concern is for your immediate protection and restoring you to a zone in which you can function.

Once you make the decision to change the pattern of your thinking, you also need to accept one very important truth: give yourself permission to accept the way you were because it served you. Be grateful to it for leading you to this new awareness.

Journal Exercise

Start to recognise some of the mental patterns or limiting beliefs present in the way you think and speak. Write down how you are feeling today and what is going on for you right now, and then go back and see if you can spot any negative mindsets that could be draining your energy. In a different-coloured pen, rewrite the sentence in a neutral or positive way and see how it shifts your energy around the statement. For example, 'my phone battery always runs out when I need it most' written from a neutral stance becomes 'phone batteries die – keep a spare battery charger in my handbag' or 'I'm always left with the jobs nobody else wants to do' to 'my role entails activities I do not enjoy'. Remember, this is not about beating yourself up but freeing yourself from any unnecessary emotional shackles that are tying you to an unrealistic and negative reality.

Coaching Exercise: Taking the Power Out of Fear

If you find yourself going over and over the same thoughts and draining away precious energy, then try this exercise to stop the cycle: have a face-to-face chat with your fear. Sound scary? Possibly not as scary as the effects of long-term denial. By denying yourself the opportunity to confront your fears you are held hostage, forced to live in inauthentic ways. It's like a web that gets bigger and more intricate the longer you ignore the spider weaving it, affecting areas of your life that are otherwise unrelated.

In your journal, write down five statements that best express your fears. You may have more or less, but aim for five. Start by clearly stating the facts or situation, and then add your response or the fearful thought attached to it. For example:

The situation	Your fear
• I don't have children	• I'm afraid I will die alone
• My daughter is an only child	• I'm afraid she will miss out and have a lonely childhood
• IVF has failed twice.	• I'm afraid it will never work and I am wasting my time and money.

Now take a look at those fears – are they as scary on paper as in your head? Probably not. You have begun to disempower them by pulling them out of the shadows of your mind.

I want you to now imagine putting on a pair of glasses that only allow you to see the truth through rational, logical and possibly comical means. You may think now is not the time for humour, but why shouldn't it be? Laughter is the best medicine and if you can crack a giggle at the absurdity of fear, then you really are sending it packing. It's fear that wants us to lie awake at night panicking, not our higher self.

Now let's look at those fears again. Take 'I don't have children and I'm afraid I will die alone,' and put on those glasses to see: 'I am surrounded by children, such as my nieces and nephews, and I have the opportunity to build beautiful, long-lasting relationships with them. I will never be alone if I allow myself to open up to their love and become their favourite aunt, who spoils them rotten.'

Or: 'My daughter is an only child and I'm afraid she will miss out and have a lonely childhood.' And now change it to: 'My daughter is loved more than she can imagine. She has every need met and we dote on her day and night. She is missing out on nothing because she has close friends and family nearby and we are strong, supportive and loving parents who provide a warm, nurturing and caring home.'

Finally: 'IVF has failed twice. I'm afraid it will never work and we are wasting our time and money.' Let it become: 'We have tried IVF twice and statistics show it sometimes takes several attempts for success. I am no different from anyone else going through these challenges and I must be patient. What if I was living in a developing country with no medical support to offer this opportunity? I am lucky I have the time and money to do this multiple times.'

When you reread your answers, hopefully you will feel more calm, confident and optimistic about your situation. By throwing water on the fire of your fear, you can see it for what it truly is − an unhelpful thought that hasn't been pulled into line. Or even if you experience a major crisis, this technique can help you handle it in a rational and logical manner. Whenever you find yourself getting overwhelmed, use this tool to anchor yourself in the facts rather than the fears.

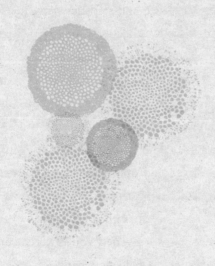

STEP 6

Releasing Control

A few swipes of your fingertip can summon up vast amounts of personal data through smart devices like iPhones, be it how many calories you consumed yesterday, the dollars sitting in your savings account, who's doing what on the other side of the planet or your Pilates class schedule. Modern-day living means more control. Control is your friend, a loyal, trusted friend that helps you thrive and make sense of this crazy world. After all, who doesn't want to be CEO of the universe? As mentioned in Step 2, your brain loves certainty and autonomy, so the more expectations you set, the more you feed your false sense of control. Unfortunately, this means the harder the wake-up call when things don't go to plan.

Obviously there is no definitive control over conception. There is nothing certain about falling pregnant. You can control how often you have sex, monitor your ovulation, take supplements and herbs – the to-do lists are endless. But ultimately you are not going to actually push that little sperm into the egg, no matter what you do. We have absolutely no control over that. All the positive thinking in the world cannot make you pregnant.

It is important to explore various avenues so that you can give trying to become pregnant your best shot. After all, one of them may actually work, in which case you can put this book down right now. Sadly, however, chances are you are still reading and you have exhausted the limits of your control. That's okay. Take it easy on yourself. It is only natural to hang on to every possibility and try to remain optimistic. Hope is an important strength to foster. It keeps the door of possibility open, even if it is only slightly ajar. But you need to be clear on how you manage control. You may not be able to realistically choose when you'll fall pregnant, but you can set a reasonable goal of pursuing every possibility of achieving a pregnancy. And this may mean handing over the control to a professional who knows a little more about biology than Dr Google. Gathering your support team is within your control and employing professionals you can trust means things are within your control even when you are having one of those self-doubting wobbly moments.

There is an easy way to distinguish healthy and unhealthy control. Thoughts that start with 'if only' are normally unhealthy, as they propose that a greater power is out there, in charge of your reality. 'If-onlys' perpetuate a sense of loss and the idea that things are outside your control. Notice how this de-energises and pulls you down? In contrast, thoughts beginning with 'I choose to' or 'my options are' put you back into the driver's seat. Even if there is nothing you can do to change a situation, you can still choose to be patient and open to hearing different suggestions.

Be kind to yourself first and foremost. Most women are self-confessed control freaks and life has served them very well with this formula. You don't get to run a successful business or head up a strategic department in an international company by trusting 'she'll be right'. The control-freak gene runs deep in your blood and causes all sorts of positive and negative effects. But you and I both know that ultimately control is only an illusion. Just watch the evening news and then tell me there is such a thing as absolute control. Roadblocks will always appear out of nowhere to challenge and bump you off course. That is the process of life, it's how we evolved as human beings, and it's a real journey that can't be mapped out in our heads.

By accepting the uncertainty of life and reframing each challenge or roadblock as part of the human experience, you can move from a space where your energy feels tight and restrictive into a state of expansion, where you are open to seeking out new possibilities and are also able to remain in a calm, balanced position where energy flows.

Letting go

Control is like a drug: it give us a sense of feeling good. It's easy to get hooked on this false sense of security. When people suffering from alcoholism decide to get sober, a successful path is the Alcoholics Anonymous Twelve-Step Program. Followers surrender control and 'believe that a Power greater than ourselves could restore us to sanity'. Believing in something greater than yourself is an opening for spirituality – God, the Divine, the Universe, Buddha, the sacred self – call it what you like, it offers insight and relief outside the reins of control. In my experience, spirituality has been the soothing balm to calm and heal the wounds of the unknown while keeping the heart open to move forward. If there is some aspect of spirituality that resonates with you, now is the time to pick up that book, listen to that speaker or just get down on your knees and pray.

Stress and control are close cousins. The more you stress, the greater the need for control. And the more you can't control, the greater the stress. I believe one way to address this toxic relationship is to get a handle on your natural stress responses, such as comfort eating or overworking, by noticing the key triggers. Awareness is key. If it's going to be a stressful week, then get prepared. You may not be able to always combat the trigger, but staying committed to a healthy routine with exercise, meditation, relaxation, massage, journalling or time in nature can boost your natural inoculation against the build-up of stress.

Redefining control within new healthy boundaries may require you to relinquish some old behaviours. Letting go of the things we cannot control can be uncomfortable at first, but remember to give yourself a pat on the back when you try it. It's a huge step just acknowledging you cannot control the planet singlehandedly. Most people would rather live in denial than face the discomfort of accepting that some things are beyond their control. You may want to do this exercise from a work perspective too. Strive to be the best version of yourself by surrendering what you cannot control and being fully present, positive and responsible for things you can. That in itself will release you from unnecessary worry and put you into a space of proactive thinking. You could add a mantra to help move through the discomfort, such as 'What will be will be, it will all work out in the end', or 'Let it be'.

Letting go of ways that no longer serve you is part of this journey. Using all you have learned to date to piece together the new and improved version of yourself is an important step in transforming this experience into an empowering one.

There's a new girl in town

Fertility issues may lead you down the existential garden path. You are no longer the old you because your comfort zone has been stretched. It's impossible to unlearn what is now your reality.

At present you may feel ill-equipped to step into the new version of yourself. It's as if you are stranded in the wilderness, wondering why everything seems different and out of control. Thoughts whip around your head as you try to make sense of this new world, and feelings can be prickly or downright overwhelming. Take comfort knowing this is exactly where you are meant to be. The wilderness is the essential stopgap on your journey. It's where you pick up new skills, knowledge and awareness about yourself and your situation that allow you to step into the new and improved version of yourself. The new you is always evolving – think how different you are now to when you were eighteen.

You are now at a fork in the road and you have a chance to direct and mould a change to your inner self. While your brain sets about getting you out of the wilderness as quickly as possible, remember that it doesn't distinguish between healthy or unhealthy thoughts, it just needs to relieve the uncomfortable sensation via the quickest neuro-pathway. If that pathway sends you down the 'grumpy old woman' route, then your brain will safely park the discomfort with the satisfaction it has done its job. While you've been steered out of the wilderness, the new you is a negative soul who finds fault with the world.

With some conscious effort, though, you can take your brain off autopilot and steer yourself through this wilderness. Using one simple command, you can choose who you want to become; instead of the grumpy old woman, tell yourself: 'There's a new girl in town. She is smart, graceful and deeply compassionate to herself. And so it is.' Upon hearing this sentence your brain will readjust its focus and actively seek out evidence and thoughts to support this mindset. But the brain is going to need constant reprogramming when in the wilderness; it's going to want to revert back to its old unhealthy ways, and it's far too exhausting to keep your mind on high alert all the time, so you need an idea for the brain to anchor to.

Coaching Exercise: Picture the New You

Enter the vision board (also known as a concept-, dream- or mood board). I'm not talking about a traditional vision board here, with random images representing your various goals, although I would heavily encourage you to create one of those too, as the physical act of sourcing images that represent your ideal life and sticking them onto a board is highly inspirational and motivating. For now I'm suggesting a piece of A4 paper or a mounted canvas – go as big as you want, but try not to go smaller than A4. This blank white space is about to become your focal point for living. This is where you consciously choose who you wish to become as a result of this fertility journey. So get scissor happy and start cutting out pictures from magazines, print off your Pinterest images or scour the internet for photos of women you admire and who hold qualities you wish to display.

Maybe your Great Aunt Betty always showed tremendous compassion for herself and others – a quality you now wish to foster and grow in yourself. But don't just stop with people, cut out words that mean something to you, values, mantras, affirmations or images of things or places – everything that represents the new empowered woman who will confidently stride away from this challenge with her head held high. Feel free to label the new you – choosing how you will refer to yourself helps fire up the pathways and makes controlling the direction of your thoughts easier.

Melissa and her partner were going through the highs and lows of infertility and every bump and shake sent tremors through their life, especially their marriage. Melissa came to coaching knowing something had to give. She allowed herself six more months and a change of approach, after which they would hang up their IVF gloves and go on a huge round-the-world holiday.

After I explained the power of vision boards, Melissa said there was only one image that she needed. It was a photo of her and her husband, Robert, having breakfast on a balcony overlooking the French Riviera. It was taken at the height of their happiness and captured why they were together and their shared love of life. Melissa kept this photo close to hand and whenever she had wobbly moments, she referred back to France and the love she felt for her partner. From this authentic sense of self, Melissa was able to get through those testing moments.

I heard from Melissa eighteen months after our sessions ended. The IVF had been unsuccessful so they went on their world holiday. Her email also included a photo of them, back on the Riviera, full of hope for the future.

'Should' versus 'Choose'

While we are designing the new you, I think it is important to leave behind harmful habits. One of the worst mental habits I find is the use of the word 'should'. I like to categorise 'should' into healthy and unhealthy: healthy refers to statements such as 'You should get out of a burning building' while unhealthy sounds something like 'You should be able to cope better than everyone else'. Both refer to a set of rules – one real, the other presumed. Since the moment you were born, rules were set upon you by parents, schoolteachers and sport coaches, to name a few. Normally, these provide a healthy framework for safe living, but when you use the word 'should' in an unhealthy and negative manner, it's as if there is an external authority greater than yourself dictating your thoughts. This creates a competing inner dialogue – what you want to do versus what you should do. Your personal power is torn. There are two instinctual ways to respond: to rebel or to succumb. If you rebel, you can resist and fight the rule but you may later be filled with guilt or remorse. Alternatively, if you reluctantly succumb, you open yourself to frustration and possible resentment. Both paths may lead to a desire to take revenge in an attempt to regain power. And when you begin to dance in the circles of revenge and power, you are susceptible to playing the victim. Power games rarely bring long-term satisfaction or fulfilment, and waste precious time and energy.

Fortunately there is a third option: conscious choice. This leaves your power intact even when you have to do something you really don't want to do. By replacing 'should' with 'choose' you are creating a sense of autonomy. For example, you may not wish to complete that report by Monday, but if you choose to work late to finish it then your actions are self-directed. This is an empowering act compared to feeling you 'should' work late to finish the report and ending up resentful at being in the office out of hours. Only you can control your response to a situation. By being open to consciously choosing your response to a situation rather than reacting to it, you automatically think more clearly and positively. It is easier to accept responsibility and consequences from this mental space.

I like to think of 'should' as a power leak and 'choose' as power fuel: one depletes your energy and keeps you stuck while the other empowers you to move on. Listen out for the word 'should' in your language. Replace any 'shoulds' with the word 'choose'. Even if it feels awkward and silly, this is a powerful habit to nurture and will soon feel like second nature.

Coaching Exercise: Own Your Vision Completely

Take a look over your vision board and notice if any of your images refer to a 'should' in your life. Did you pick a specific image because you felt you should want or be that? Ask yourself where this idea comes from. Is it something that will add greater meaning, joy and fulfilment to your life? If not, feel free to change the image to something more authentic.

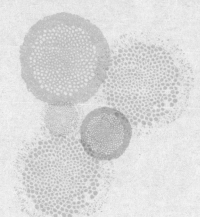

STEP 7

Building Your
Emotional Toolkit

R emember the idea of the wilderness, the time when you are no longer the old you but not yet fully the new you? After the vision board exercise you will have the new you in sight, but what do you do while you wait for this person to take her seat? Old habits, mindsets and fears can all come out to play when you least expect them. These may sabotage your effort and send you on a downhill spiral where it's one step forward but three steps back. This is bound to happen – you are human and your brain is designed to flee back to your comfort zone. Better the devil you know, right?

You need tools while you're in this wilderness. You wouldn't begin to climb Mount Everest without the adequate equipment, yet so often we venture into new challenging mental terrain with no toolkit to hand. This step is all about building your emotional toolkit, not just for this journey but for the rest of your life. Think of it as a first-aid kit for your soul. But before you can apply the first-aid kit you need to know the injury, so to speak. It would be a lot easier if you could identify broken thoughts or bleeding emotions and simply apply the appropriate dressing. When you are dealing with that tricky machine upstairs you need to outsmart your brain's deceptive programming.

I think the cleverest way to do this is to become very familiar with the types of thoughts that take you away from your higher self or the new you, and label them so that you can catch and categorise them before they commence their destructive ways. In the case study in Step 5, Sally was describing her inner self as a 'crazy monkey'. Buddhism also refers to the idea of having a monkey mindset, as if there are loose monkeys in the office (your head) or a lunatic in the attic. The idea is that there is an untrained and slightly unhinged being sitting in the control seat of your brain rather than your higher self.

Throughout my experience working with women, I have seen many 'crazy monkeys'. Infertility seems to specifically bring out the big five false-thinking godfathers of the monkey family: blame, shame, guilt, regret and perfectionism. And each monkey has its own way of bringing you down.

Blame monkey: My doctor should have told me more; that nurse was useless.

Shame monkey: I'm so embarrassed and belittled by this whole IVF process. Why can't I be normal?

Guilt monkey: It's all my fault because I have left it too
late to start a family.

Regret monkey: Why didn't we try sooner?

Perfectionism monkey: Everything has to be done
properly or I just won't bother.

Perfectionism is the King Kong of the monkeys. Rarely is any area of life exempt from this form of self-sabotage. When this monkey takes the wheel, it whispers the tunes of dissatisfaction and unrealistic expectations into your ear, so you are rarely able to meet your own standards and, consequently, become unaccepting of yourself. This can transpire from home to work to health and all the other areas of your life.

If you can identify with any of these particular monkeys or if you have another monkey on your back, then it's essential to spend a moment jotting down exactly what you are dealing with. The more familiar you become with your monkey, the less likely it is going to be able to slip past your attention and get out. Clients have described everything from an angry teenage monkey wearing goth attire to green creatures resembling the Hulk. Knowing some of the trademark statements your monkey likes to repeat – such as 'It's all your fault' – can help you catch the beast before it runs amok. Once you notice the monkey activated in your thinking, just call it what it is: 'There goes my blame monkey again', or 'Hello, regret monkey, I see you!'

It's important that you start to notice and act upon the divide in your thinking. Your higher self, your vision-board image, needs to be calling the shots around here, not your lower self. The monkeys are just a representation of your lower self that you don't have to listen to. As real as it may feel and as compelling and even addictive as it may seem to act upon the thoughts and impulses of your lower self, they are just thoughts and you can choose where to focus your attention and behave accordingly. Wherever you place your attention is what you are hardwiring into your brain, which means repeated use will create a habit. To become the new and empowered version of yourself, you need to put your focused attention on the thoughts that are in alignment with your higher self. Over time you will become that person because you are directing those empowering habits to your brain.

The trick is to know how to handle one of the monkeys once you have caught it. This is where you call upon your emotional toolkit. During a monkey siege you are not going to be able to think very clearly, so don't rely upon your higher self to get you out of the jam straightaway. You are simply going to pick one of the actions on your emotional toolkit list to keep your mind distracted with a healthy and positive activity while the intensity of the monkey's grip loosens. By committing to an action from your toolkit, you can focus on a healthy distraction that will eventually lead you to a more balanced and even keel – where you can go about your business and get back to normal.

You could:

- Drink some water
- Take a brisk walk, preferably in a natural environment
- Call a friend
- Complete a quick meditation
- Take ten deep breaths
- Watch some comedy and laugh
- Turn on some bubblegum TV shows, the light-hearted stuff
- Knit, paint, sew, bake, plant – anything that gets the creative juices flowing
- Listen to music – create a pick-me-up playlist for these emergencies
- Spend time with your pet
- Exercise
- Repeat an affirmation (see Coaching Exercise: Positive Affirmations on page 82 for examples)
- Listen to a podcast or something inspirational.

Write out at least five strategies for your emotional toolkit and place the list somewhere you can access it quickly, like on the fridge or in your handbag. Remember, you must go straight to one of these tools when you are feeling the effects of a monkey in play. Don't question it, don't think about it, don't analyse it, just do it, and keep doing it until the strong emotions have passed. Enrol your partner if you feel comfortable enough to share. No doubt they will have some monkeys running around upstairs too and may benefit from the exercise as well.

Tracey was an incredibly gifted artist. During an early coaching session, she discovered a tea party of monkeys when reflecting upon a dilemma. She dedicated an afternoon to painting each monkey and then wrote a poem to describe their characteristics in full. This cathartic exercise proved very amusing, but also heightened her awareness of her damaging thoughts. Of course the monkeys did not disappear and from time to time she was still plagued by them, but she recognised them for what they were and knew what to do about them.

Coaching Exercise: Positive Affirmations

To ensure the best possible experience during any fertility treatment, you need to have productive and self-serving thoughts. You can't control the end result, but you can control your response to it. By investing time in the daily practice of positive affirmations, you are taking control of your mind, doing everything you can to stop those rogue worries or detrimental thoughts roaming around your head unchecked. Your fertility experience is far too important to allow negative, out-of-control mind chatter to sabotage you. Command your reality by focusing your thoughts on what you want, not what you don't want.

Try using some of the affirmations below or create your own list. Repeat one or more statements ten times every morning and throughout your day, or whenever you find negative thoughts creeping in. This will help you keep positive and focused. If it helps, write the affirmations on little cards and keep them close to hand. Stick them on your mirror so you repeat them when you brush your hair, or on the fridge, or even as reminders that pop up on your phone.

- *I trust in the process and in my body.*
- *I am calm, peaceful and relaxed.*
- *Solutions to challenges come easily to me.*
- *I find the positive in all circumstances.*
- *I find strength in my vulnerability.*
- *I graciously accept my life.*
- *I am a well of patience and calm.*
- *My body is my friend and ally.*
- *I seek to create the positive from the negative.*
- *I am grateful for my body.*
- *I love my body and accept it wholly.*

- *I nurture my body to be the best it can be.*
- *I surround myself with loving and supportive people.*
- *I am worthy of happiness and love.*
- *I feel supported and loved on my fertility journey.*
- *I confidently speak my mind.*
- *I release all anxious thoughts.*
- *I know my partner loves and supports me.*
- *I fill my mind only with constructive and productive thoughts.*
- *I confidently ask for and receive help when I need it.*
- *I allow myself to feel my emotions and then let them pass.*

Coaching Exercise: Saying No

One of the biggest gifts you can learn to give yourself is the magic of the word 'no'. Saying no to others sometimes means saying yes to you. But saying no is hard and most people would rather say yes to avoid embarrassment, guilt or letting someone down. It's easier to deal with our own disappointment than know we caused someone else's. Sometimes we just need to learn the specific language of how to say no to be free from over-committing ourselves. Here are some things to remember:

- Saying yes to yourself is as important as saying yes to others. Value your time and energy.

- If you say no, you buy yourself a precious commodity – time. Use it to see family and friends or spending time doing something you value and that brings you joy.
- See yourself as assertive and responsible for your time and energy. Protect it with the occasional 'no'.
- To avoid conflict, practise a set response to buy yourself time to think, such as 'I need to check my calendar', or 'Can I get back to you tomorrow?'
- Do you really want to say yes? Does your intuition agree with you? Listen to your higher self for guidance.
- Find a comfortable sentence that kindly and respectfully says no, such as 'I'm really sorry I can't help this time.'
- Acknowledge every time you successfully say yes to yourself and soon it will become second nature.

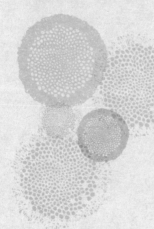

STEP 8

Handling Family
and Friends

Elouise, a single woman, had three rounds of unsuccessful IVF in two years. Her group of friends had given birth to five babies in that time. Although Elouise reported feeling torn with jealousy and guilt toward their growing families, she also held on to the belief that those babies were not meant for her. Elouise remembers how social gatherings were always awkward: 'They don't want me to feel sad hearing about their babies or cause me more pain, and I really do want to be part of their life. But it's like rubbing salt in a wound.' Elouise found herself withdrawing from her friends and receiving fewer invitations to events. Instead of dwelling on the isolation she decided to have an honest conversation with two of her best friends about how they could support her as well as reaffirm the importance of the friendship.

Many women feel their fertility experience affects their relationship with friends and family because of the unspoken elephant in the room. Of course you want to be a good friend and share in their joy, but it can be hard to listen to new mothers discuss reflux dramas when they are holding a precious baby in their arms. It's totally normal to have conflicting emotions in these kinds of situations. Uncharitable or negative thoughts, or what you can now call those crazy monkeys, are natural. Even the most compassionate and loving person isn't a saint under extreme stress. Just because you feel jealousy doesn't mean you're a bad person, it makes you a real human being. Holding yourself back or withdrawing from the full engagement of your friendships, as Elouise did, can often feel like a safe way to operate. And that is totally fine. Give yourself permission to do what you need to do to keep functioning. Remember not to judge your emotions or thoughts as they are just the transient states of the monkeys and you know they will eventually pass. Do not attach yourself to any labels. It's tempting to formulate an identity based on how you're feeling in the moment, but it's not the truth about who you are. You are much bigger than one type of emotional expression or thought. Look at your vision board. Reconnect to the real you. If still in doubt, ask those who care about you to remind you of all your strengths and quality traits so you can get back to the core of yourself and remember the vast complexity that is you, your unique history, your present moment and your future possibilities.

However, when you withdraw from friends and family you can potentially send conflicting messages, especially if they don't know what's going on inside your head. Without breaching your privacy, you may need to reaffirm specific relationships by letting them know you need some space. This can be via text, letter, email or over a cup of tea. It is totally acceptable to decline invitations to any social events at this time. It will give you greater peace of mind to know your friends and family are aware how important they are to you, but also that you need some space right now.

Sometimes well-meaning friends or family members say things that hurt – really hurt. As much as you may have to remind yourself they mean well and are just worried about you, such moments can add unnecessary burdens to your already heavy shoulders. One useful way to avoid this is by providing loved ones with a structure of how you need to be handled at this time – presuming they know how to read your mind or even have the skills to say the right thing is setting up the relationship for failure. Of course, this is all new to you too and no one is expecting you to be able to deal with the repercussions of others experiencing your pain. However, the following outline may assist in preparing for a conversation with those you care about.

Family and friends help sheet

Please acknowledge my emotional range and the fact I don't have control over it:

Sad – Hopeless – Angry – Scared – Resentful – Stressed out – Ashamed – Out of control – Useless – Outraged – Bitter – Despairing – Defensive – Full of blame

Ways you can help:

1. Validate my feelings.
   a. You can't take away my pain.
   b. Please don't say you can imagine it.
   c. Just knowing you are accepting me as I am helps.
2. Listen to me.
   a. Supportively and sensitively.
   b. Patiently and without judgement.
3. Understand the process.
   a. It's natural to not want to socialise.
   b. Even though I may withdraw, it's not personal.
   c. You are still important to me.
   d. This experience is really emotionally challenging and hard.
4. Drop expectations.
   a. Please don't expect me to be my normal self right now.
   b. I may not attend certain events.
   c. I'm not being self-indulgent or overreacting, I'm focusing on self-care and self-management the best way I know how.
5. Ways to support me.
   a. Please be there if I want to talk.
   b. Consider taking me to a meal, a cinema, or other distractions.
   c. Don't talk about your children.
   d. Give me private notice of pregnancy announcements.
   e. Don't assume anything, please ask.

It may not be appropriate to hand this information over to everyone in your life as there are different levels of intimacy and closeness in your family and friendship circles. Call upon specific friends for their listening ear and others for an afternoon of fun. Everyone brings different strengths to the table, so pick and choose who can best support you in different ways.

When dealing with someone who is in your outer circle, remember you do not owe them an explanation. Chances are they have a little more courage than those closer to you to ask prying and insensitive questions. Have a list of at least three standard replies that you can deliver in any situation with little emotional attachment. You have every right to protect your boundaries. It may be wise to choose to deliver a standard line rather than give that person a piece of your mind – your energy is best reserved for more worthy causes.

Here are some examples of answers to the standard question, 'So when are you two going to start a family?'

- When the time is right.
- That's not something I can answer right now.
- Why do you want to know?

You can always add some humour to lighten the mood:

- When they come with a guarantee.
- Why, are you selling yours?

Quickly change the subject back to them, something like, 'How is your work/holiday/new home?' Alternatively, you can pretend you didn't hear the question and just carry on. If they don't get the hint, excuse yourself from the conversation.

Coaching Exercise: Strengthen Your Comebacks

Practice is the key to delivering a powerful and yet calm comeback to enquiries from family and friends. Set some time aside to brainstorm all the possible triggers you could encounter or have encountered with family and friends. When you have your list of potential inflammatory statements, I want you to write your cool, calm and collected responses. Script all the potential scenarios and be very clear on your comebacks. Enrol your partner too as he or she will benefit from the preparation.

Now role-play the scene either with your partner, a trusted friend or a mirror. The more uncomfortable you feel saying your chosen comeback, the more you must practise. This will become natural over time. By building confidence in your comebacks, you will become less stressed at social events and free yourself from anticipating the comments.

STEP 9

Relationship
Bumps

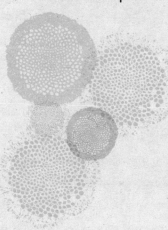

STEP

Relationship
Bumps

Every relationship will weather the storm of infertility differently. I have seen couples who have a strong and deep understanding of each other travel to hell and back under the strains of infertility, and others who casually take it in their stride. It's normal to expect some relationship stress, the degree of which will depend on the dynamics of the individuals and the communication structures in place. It seems this experience can deepen existing cracks in a relationship. This is not bad news, as it means issues that may have remained unresolved and festering for years can now be consciously healed with the right care and attention. Couples who experience infertility usually learn coping strategies that equip them for a long and happy life together. A relationship isn't truly a relationship until it has been tested.

A golden rule for surviving those stressful days is the 'Twenty-Minute Rule': limit your fertility talk to just twenty minutes a day, unless you have new information to discuss. This will help you both become more specific and succinct in your communication. Because time is limited, each of you will have to deliver your message as clearly and quickly as possible – meaning you both need to listen intently and commit fully to the conversation. Knowing it's only twenty minutes means things won't drag on all day or night and the rest of your time is free to get on with other aspects of life. I suggest setting an alarm and not getting too comfortable, maybe using the spare room or kitchen table to talk, not the lounge or bedroom.

You are both totally unique individuals with completely different brains. Even though you may finish each other's sentences and 'know' what the other one is thinking, it's worth taking some time out to explore and understand how you each process stress. Knowing yourself and your personality traits and recognising specific triggers help detect unconstructive filters in your thinking. By thinking beyond your agenda it's easier to truly empathise and express compassion to your loved one. Listen to each other without judgement or offering unrequested solutions. To hear and validate each other's journey is incredibly healing and powerful.

There are two words I recommend you remove from your communication: 'why' and 'you'. Both subconsciously point the blaming finger and automatically raise defences. Try to state things objectively and replace 'why' with 'what', 'when', 'how' or 'where'. For example, instead of 'Why do you always do that?' try 'How can this be done differently from now on?'

If you are an outgoing and social person, and like to consider multiple pieces of information at the same time, but your partner is more quiet and introverted, be respectful of his or her need to process information slowly and thoroughly, one issue at a time. Patience is the key: both partners will need to progress at the rate of the slower partner. This can be the Achilles' heel of communication. If things deteriorate despite your best efforts, immediately seek out professional help – what may seem a colossal mountain for the two of you can usually be deconstructed into molehills by a professional simply by reframing the message.

A wonderful resource is Gary Chapman's book *The Five Love Languages*. He details five different ways of expressing love in a relationship. Speaking your partner's love language amplifies the feelings of closeness and appreciation between you, not to mention love. It's also great to be able to clearly articulate your needs in black-and-white facts.

Here are three things to consider in your relationship:

1. How can you keep your communication open and honest during this time?
    a. Schedule a date night.
    b. Consider writing down how you are feeling instead of verbalising it.

c. Use the skills of a trained professional to help overcome stubborn obstacles in your relationship.

2. Have a resentment check-in. It's easy to find resentments unintentionally building up.

   a. Write a list of all the niggling things that are currently annoying you in your relationship.

   b. Re-examine them with a critical eye. How important are these right now?

   c. Can you let them go and focus on the greater good or do you need to do something about this?

   d. Keep a list of the common resentments you find and stick it on the fridge. For example, your partner keeps leaving the coffee machine for you to clean even though you don't drink coffee. When a resentment becomes apparent, call it for what it is and clear the space between the two of you.

3. Keep a love jar. It's very important to keep the reasons you are together at the forefront of your mind. This person is your life partner and source of love.

   a. Get a large glass jar and fill it with love notes for each other. Choose a colour to represent each person and write out reasons why you love the other or things you would like to do together.

   b. Each morning start your day with a new note of love or activity to integrate into your week.

No matter where this journey takes you, remember why you are here. Love needs to be the core of your motivation and intentions within your relationship. Remember, this solid foundation of love can weather the roughest of storms.

Claudia and Mike were two peas in a pod; they even had the same personality test results. Although my coaching was only with Claudia, their relationship was a primary topic in our conversations. Despite the tumultuous nature of their relationship, there was a deep love and commitment to be together. Frequent arguments resulted in childlike behaviour as neither wanted to be wrong. Their repeated IVF cycles had worn away Claudia's self-confidence and eventually she recognised her desperate need for a break. During this time we worked together to uncover a new way for her to communicate with Mike. Claudia started to own her needs and by making some subtle adjustments to their language, the inherent conflict within started to subside. This meant the surrender of their petulant score cards, an acceptance of each other's needs and recognition of their similar discomfort with being wrong and their need to be right.

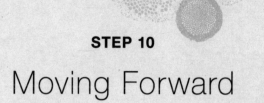

STEP 10

Moving Forward

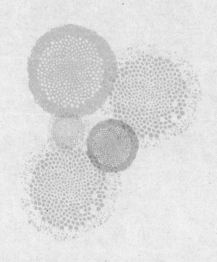

A nd so here you are, moving forward. The hardest part is over once the decision to seek help from a fertility specialist has been made. It doesn't mean you have to do anything specific, like start a radical detox diet or begin IVF, it means you are going to ask for assistance in understanding what's not working, one step at a time. Rome wasn't built in a day and all those old chestnuts. But it's true. Moving forward means you place one foot in front of the other and just keep going; you are moving closer to a greater understanding of what's going on. There is a wonderful saying about driving in the dark: you can only see as far as the headlights shine but you keep driving with the faith the road will keep revealing itself. And that is how you need to think now – keep faith that you are moving forward with the confidence and strength to hear the facts, assess the data and evaluate your situation.

Remember, facts are more empowering than fiction, so challenge yourself to confidently move forward knowing you can trust yourself to ask the right questions, challenge any unhelpful thinking and allow whatever needs to happen to just happen. Chances are you will not recognise the strength in your vulnerability, the courage in your confusion or the openness in your fragility until you look back one day and smile. It's hard living with uncertainty, but I know you can do it. We don't know our capacity until we are genuinely tested.

The first person to talk to is normally your GP, for a referral letter to a fertility specialist. Many first-time patients report a deep sense of relief after attending their first meeting with an IVF doctor. As opposed to surrendering their power, they feel they are back in control, heading toward a solution. Many doors will open when you make the decision to move forward. Choosing the right process for you and your partner means a return to the drawing board and navigating the facts. This can also be true for exploring egg/sperm donation or adoption paths. If egg or sperm donation is your next step to starting a family, you will need to understand the new language and requirements for donation. New terminology and rules regarding the process will require time and patience to learn. The same stands for the adoption process. Depending on your country of residence, laws and processes are different. You may even need to travel overseas to achieve your goal.

To confidently move forward, here are some things to consider:

1. Use a large folder to store all the relevant documents and information you gather in one central location.
2. Allocate specific time with your partner to process the data.
3. Draw a plan of action so you know each step required to proceed in the directions available to you (see Coaching Exercise below).

Book appointments even if you haven't completely made up your minds on how to proceed – there is no harm in gathering as much information as possible and noticing how you feel as you venture down each path.

Remember, inaction is closely followed by anxiety. By moving forward one step at a time you are getting closer to a solution and keeping anxiety at bay.

On page 147 you will find a resource called 'The IVF Cycle Handbook', which is specifically written as a coaching companion to an IVF cycle.

Coaching Exercise: MAP your MOVE

Structure your next step forward as if it were a business plan. This keeps your thinking constructive and practical. With fertility in mind, I created MAP your MOVE as an adaptation on the traditional SMART (Specific, Measureable, Attainable, Realistic, Time frame) goal model.

M	Measurable
A	Achievable
P	Positive – focus and time frame

M	Momentum
O	Obstacles
V	Visualisation
E	Engage

Once you have decided your goal or intention (IVF, egg or sperm donation, adoption or another path to parenthood), write it down. You may wish to work with an intention because it is more fluid than a rigid goal. Intentions foster adaptability and flexibility by adapting to obstacles along the way. Then MAP it out.

For example:

INTENTION: USE AN EGG DONOR

M – Measurable:

1. How much information do I need to gather before I can make an informed decision?

2. Who is on my professional support team? For example, doctors, counsellors, agencies.

3. How many attempts will we consider?

4. How much money will we spend on this?

A – Achievable:

1. What are the medical facts to take into consideration?
2. What is working in our favour?
3. What is working against us?
4. How do our finances fare against the cost?

P – Positive focus and time frame:

1. What is the positive focus I need to remember when times are tough?
2. How much time are we going to allocate to this?
3. We will work toward a Reassess Date of [insert date] if things are not working out.

Once you have mapped out your goal or intention, it's time to jump into action with MOVE.

M – Momentum

1. Break down the intention into mini goals.
2. Under each mini goal write out the monthly, weekly and daily actions needed.
3. Commit to each action by allocating a specific time and date.
4. Lock the actions into your calendar, set alarms, enrol friends, anything to keep you accountable.
5. If you fail to complete an action, move it to another time. Don't let it slide.

O – Obstacles

1. Contemplate every possible challenge, resistance or roadblock.
2. Get clear on how to overcome these obstacles.
3. Be prepared as much as possible.

V – Vision

When the days get wearying, you will need an inspiring vision to keep you motivated. Having a visual representation can stir emotions and reignite your commitment. Find a symbol, image, saying, object or anything that represents your intention and keep it in sight.

E – Engage

1. Gather your support crew. For example, doctors, health professionals, case agents, etc.
2. Ensure you have confidence in each of your crew members.
3. Call upon family and friends who can assist you at this time.

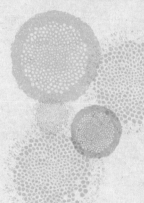

STEP 11

When Enough
Is Enough

Reaching the decision to stop fertility treatment is not easy, but then what has been on this journey? It's a huge issue to address and something you may wish to begin to explore before you are actually at the point of making a forced decision. Remember, the brain loves certainty and if you can set the expectation of how many cycles or months you will commit to the process, then your brain can concentrate on the task at hand rather than have a random uncertainty monkey periodically making an appearance in your thought process.

Everyone's circumstances are totally unique. There are many important aspects, both physically and emotionally, that need to be taken into consideration in understanding when to stop trying for a baby. While some women choose to undertake only one round of IVF, others may decide, say, eleven is their limit. Some couples receive medical advice to stop or find the physical intervention too hard to bear, while others find the financial strain or other life priorities are the catalyst to cease treatment.

When deliberating over the good and bad reasons to end treatment I have heard a variety of reasons I would categorise as 'band aid' decisions. These stem from a need to avoid the pain of decision-making in the moment, with little consideration for any possible future needs. It's understandable to want to end the suffering but decisions made in haste are often bad decisions for the future.

Here are a collection of detrimental thoughts or monkeys to be aware of:

- Disappointment monkey – worrying you will let your doctor, acupuncturist or support team down.
- False-hope monkey – telling you to take 'just one more cycle'.
- Don't-be-a-wimp monkey – stopping now would be a sign of weakness and failure.
- Surrender monkey – it's all too hard and needs to stop now.

One of the more deceptive thought processes I have encountered is the incessant hunt for the perfect doctor – someone who showers you with promises, reassurances and success rates. They basically tell you all you long to hear, when really the truth of the situation is in front of you. It can be another means of avoiding the decision-making process.

This decision could be the toughest you ever have to make. Your logical self may know that stopping is the right thing to do, but just as you feel the decision has been made, a sense of hope often fires up and upsets all logic by throwing in self-doubt and hesitation for good measure. Finding your own way to reach the decision to stop is extremely important. This is a decision that you and your partner will carry for the rest of your life. How you decide to close this chapter of your lives can influence the start of the next one.

You have two internal allies in making this decision: your rational brain (monkeys aside) and your intuition. The former is there to provide the structure to precisely discern all the facts, while your intuition provides the subtle insights to guide you toward your best outcome.

Coaching Exercise: Fact Feeler

Let's start with your rational brain. Firstly, gather all the facts. Be clear on the financial costs, time costs, opportunity costs and physical costs you have paid with each cycle and how they will affect you if you do another one. Examples of the opportunity costs include declining a promotion at work, postponing a new business venture or holiday, or being able to care for elderly parents. It might be useful to categorise each area under the following headings: financial, emotional, social, psychological, relationship, time, opportunity, physical – you can add any other heading you find appropriate.

Now you have a clear picture of the past and future factors, using the table below as an example, rank on a scale of 1 to 10 (with 10 being the most positive score) how comfortable you are right now to carry the impact of another round of treatment. A score over 5 would possibly indicate a strong desire to keep going while anything below may indicate it's time to stop. Tally up your marks for an overall score out of 80. A score lower than 40 would be a clear indication it may be time to stop while a score above 50 would suggest you may have a stronger case for considering a new cycle. Are there some areas of consideration that weigh greater than others? How did they score? Try giving this exercise to your partner and schedule a time to review your answers together. Being able to openly and honestly communicate how you feel is an absolute must for you both to find the confidence and peace in your final decision.

This example came from Cathy, who had just finished her third cycle when she did this exercise:

Key areas of consideration	Facts and feelings	
Financial	$14,000 spent to date. Need to re-mortgage to do again, stressful to have used up our savings, no buffer if we lose our jobs. Uncomfortable with financial uncertainty caused by re-mortgaging.	3/10
Emotional	Really hard to handle, hate the futility, feelings of frustration and not sure I can handle another disappointment. But still feel that flicker of hope.	2/10

Key areas of consideration	Facts and feelings	
Social	Not been able to socialise much, taking its toll on friends as I'm never there, sick of deflecting questions. Christmas is around the corner and not sure I want to be going through a round when everyone visits.	5/10
Psychological	Felt crazy most of the time but Dr was really helpful as was forum so feel more supported than during first cycle. Know what to expect now.	7/10
Relationship	Separate bedrooms, hard to talk to him, he doesn't really appreciate how much I have to sacrifice. Not sure how much he wants this anymore.	2/10
Time	Time away from work but they have been great and understanding. No real time cost other than tests etc. Just my biological clock ticking, making me stressed.	5/10
Opportunity	We haven't had a holiday for two years now. Both really tired and depleted. If I keep avoiding promotion at work then they may think I am not interested in growing my career. I need my career.	2/10
Physical	Put on 8 kilos since started and feel really unhealthy, would love to get back into my exercise and feel normal again, and never have to push another needle into my skin.	2/10

Because Cathy scored 28/80, she felt a deep sadness, but also a small sense of hope that she could begin to think of what they could do to move on as opposed to the sense of limbo that haunted them. After completing the exercise, Cathy was able to clearly see in facts and figures how she felt about investing in another cycle. It gave her the confidence to own her feelings and clearly articulate her thoughts to her husband.

Turning on intuition

Now you have a clear picture of the facts, it's time to tune into your intuition. As I have previously mentioned, it is not easy to trust your higher self at this time due to the artificial hormones, extreme emotional swings and all the other triggers buried deep inside, but hopefully your intuition is there whispering words of wisdom. Connecting to your mind's insights can be hard if you lead a busy life. Go for a nature walk or a walk along the beach, take a holiday or schedule some time out to quieten the noise and distraction around you so you can literally ask yourself what you think and feel about the decision intuitively. Give yourself a time frame to actually trial a decision – this can bring new feelings or thoughts to the surface. For example, give yourself one month to think about childfree living. Guide all your thoughts and feelings to this and see what comes up for you while you trial the scenario. Enlist your partner too. If a month seems too short, then think for as long as necessary until you gather all the available insights from this potential reality.

When the decision is finally reached, in with the anger and confusion a sense of relief and control is often waiting to surface. You can now stop the limbo. The realisation it is now possible to start redesigning your life may not come immediately, though, as there are many mixed emotions to process first. It is normal to feel anger, grief, despair – you name it. These emotions may even get misdirected towards your nurses, doctors or those close to you. Remember to give yourself a break – nobody is perfect under fire. These people are your support team and understand the stress, but for your own peace of mind, try to balance the intensity of your emotions with time out for you. Give yourself time to calm down, regroup and regain balance.

If the door to IVF begins to close it may signal the opportunity for another to open. The decision to end medical intervention does not necessarily mean the end of the possibility of raising a family. Further options may include adoption, fostering or returning to the medical drawing boards for egg, sperm or embryo donation. But venturing down the path of non-genetic parenthood requires the healing of the broken dream of having your own biological child. Grief is an inevitable step in moving forward, one that cannot be avoided. If non-biological parenthood is an option for you both, then I would encourage you to use the Fact Feeler exercise on page 115 to determine how you each feel about this option. Then it is all about again gathering information and building your support team and resources around you to make it happen. I recommend speaking to a professional counsellor or therapist who specialises in the fields of donation, adoption or fostering.

The passage of grief

Grief in the traditional sense is the loss of someone or something important to you. The first thing I learned when training to be a counsellor was the complexity of grief. Grief does not fit into an orderly box. Someone grieving the loss of their mother may find it easier to cope than someone losing their beloved cat. We all experience loss differently, and knowing that no two brains are the same obviously means we cannot force ourselves or others through the grieving process. Your partner may grieve very differently from you and they are perfectly within their rights to do whatever it takes to get themselves through this painful time, just as you too must give yourself permission to fully experience the process with no judgements, labels or expectations. You need to mourn the bereavement of your hopes and dreams – just because you don't have a physical family doesn't mean you haven't spent a lifetime thinking and planning for one. Mourning the death of your dream to become a parent is your human right and a critical step toward healing.

In 1969, American psychiatrist Elizabeth Kübler-Ross detailed the five stages of grief in her book *On Death and Dying*. Although these stages are common and, to a certain degree, universal, they are not a linear process from start to finish, especially when it comes to fertility grief. There may be a specific loss, such as a miscarriage, that triggers the grief, or possibly it began with the words 'fertility problems'. With few clear boundaries to this process, it's safe to say you must take from the five stages what helps normalise and rationalise your experience of infertility.

Here are the traditional stages of grief through the lens of infertility:

Denial

- Disbelief that it's actually happening to you.

- Relying on hope as opposed to facts.

- Expecting a lab error or incorrect samples to explain the results.

- Saying everything is okay and you are not actually upset.

- Immediately starting another IVF cycle or finding a new doctor to keep distracted from the emotional pain.

- Denial actually helps you deal with the gravity of the situation, and by filtering reality in stages it helps protect your sense of identity as it integrates your new circumstances.

Anger

- As denial passes anger may appear as outrage at the injustice of the situation. 'It's not fair', 'Why me?', 'She drinks and smokes and still falls pregnant' and 'It's all your fault' are some common expressions of this anger.

- You may find yourself directing the anger toward parents, pregnant women or family members for no rational reason.

- Being angry at your medical team or health professional is also common as anger likes to find a target.
- The intensity of anger will eventually pass but it's important to express and identify the emotions as they appear in order to get them out of your system.

Bargaining

- Thinking you can bargain your way into success by making promises such as to be happy for the next pregnant person you meet, being a nicer person or giving more to charity.
- Setting unrealistic expectations to follow a specific diet, lifestyle changes and whatever drastic measures are suggested to you.
- Thinking you may jinx yourself if you don't follow through on promises or bargains you make with yourself.

Depression

- Feeling a deep well of sadness and isolation.
- Finding yourself frequently crying throughout the day or night.
- Feeling alone because no one understands.
- Loss of hope replaced with despair: 'We will never become parents so what's the point of trying?'
- Lack of interest in normally enjoyable activities.
- Your sleep or eating patterns may become disrupted.

- If this phase seems too overwhelming or has gone on for a long period of time you may benefit from speaking to a professional therapist to help navigate your way to acceptance.

Acceptance

- Hearing yourself say 'We will be okay', 'I will be okay' or 'We will get through this'.
- Feeling a growing sense of ownership over your life and how you want to live.
- Beginning to set goals or explore alternative options such as egg or sperm donation, or adoption.
- Allowing yourself to constructively think about life without children and what that looks like.

Remember, coping with the loss of your baby dream is a totally unique and private process. Research says it can take up to two years to fully process grief. Go at your own speed and remain open and honest with your partner as well as yourself. You both have to establish a new equilibrium for living, and to achieve this there will be much unpredictability as the emotional balance begins to restore. Be kind to yourself and to your partner while things settle down. Remember to use the professional services of therapists to assist you if you need a little help.

I once heard grief described as a black box – deep, dark and undisguisable. The black box is filled with the grief of loss. It's never to be taken away or forgotten. It can burst its lid and overflow at any point with no warning. It's something that travels with us no matter where we go. The black box needs to be honoured as it is now part of the rich tapestry of your history. In time, it will weave into the complexity of your life experience as you rebuild your world around it. Part of who you are and what you now do with your life will stem from having it with you.

The steep learning curve you have endured may in time reveal itself as a hidden blessing, providing new strengths and skills, more profound relationships or deeper compassion toward others. As acceptance settles, your imagination opens for a new version of life to rush in and take hold. Opportunities such as career development, travel, stronger relationships or a sense of purpose or calling may unfold, pointing you in the direction of previously uncharted territory. When we move beyond resistance, life can reveal exciting new plans.

Coaching Exercise: Getting through Grief with Mindfulness

If you haven't already got the message, let me state it one more time: you need to be kind to yourself. Self-compassion is not some sweet notion; it is scientifically proven to increase general wellbeing and relationships, not to mention the reported decrease in anxiety and depression. Self-compassion is different to self-esteem. The former builds on a deep acceptance of oneself without comparison to others or condemnation of self. It focuses on being kind, loving and understanding, despite the obstacle or failures experienced. Self-esteem, in contrast, can set a competitive bar between you and others and bases self-worth on how well you compare. There is often judgement of others and self in the continuous race to being special.

Here are some suggestions to build your self-compassion:

- Give your body the message that it's important and deserves nurturing.
    - Eat healthily.
    - Exercise just enough for your energy levels in the moment.
    - Have a massage, facial, pedicure – anything that makes you feel pampered.
    - Buy clothes that make you feel amazing.
    - Invest in comfortable relaxation clothes for evenings at home. Don't underestimate the power of super-comfy slippers, trackie daks and a hoodie. They feel heavenly after a day of work clothes and send the message to your body to relax.
- Journal once a day as a healthy exercise to access your feelings – they need nurturing too. Leave blame, shame or judgement at the door.
- Write a letter to yourself (or whoever in your life you need to) offering forgiveness and acceptance to release negative feelings.

- Set up a ritual, such as lighting a candle, to symbolise the processing of grief. It could be an unspoken act between you and your partner to light the candle when strong emotions are present but you don't feel like talking about them.

Find a support group. Evidence suggests connecting to others with a similar experience aids the healing process.

Finally, a daily practice of mindfulness is a fantastic way of developing greater wellbeing. Mindfulness is the art of focusing your attention on the present moment with acceptance and non-judgement. By keeping in the present moment you are releasing your attention from future worries and past regrets. There is evidence that consciously living in the moment leads to improved health, increased states of happiness and enhanced capacity to handle adversity.

Before all mindfulness exercises you must first make yourself comfortable, loosen any tight clothing, take off uncomfortable shoes and place your feet flat on the ground or sit cross-legged on a cushion on the floor. Take yourself away from any distracting people and turn technology off. If you are concerned about time, set an alarm so you know exactly when your five, ten or thirty minutes are up. Closing your eyes can also improve your experience.

Following are three basic mindfulness exercises:

The breath: Inhale deeply, focusing purely on the sensation of the air entering your nostrils. Don't worry about your stomach or chest rising and falling, just focus on the feeling of the air entering and leaving your nostrils. Now breathe in to the count of one and breathe out to the count of two, breathe in to the count of three and out to the count of four, and so on. Count all the way to ten then start over again.

If you lose count just return to one and start again. Witness your inner world meeting your outer world. Consider each passing thought as a cloud in the sky. You are the entire vast blue sky, and these clouds are just floating past. Know you are more than the clouds, detach yourself from them and let them pass.

This may feel like eternity if you have a busy mind. Even more reason to keep practising. If your mind wanders, don't think about it or question it or beat yourself up – escort it back to your breathing and go back to the count of one.

The chocolate: Take a small piece of chocolate. Hold the wrapper in your hand, notice how it feels. Look at the chocolate as you unwrap it: notice the colour, let your eyes examine all aspects of it. Inhale the aroma. Place the chocolate on your tongue and just hold it there. Notice the need to chew it, notice the different flavours. If your mind wanders, bring it back to the chocolate. Let it melt in your mouth, examine the texture, taste, smell, weight, size – explore everything about the chocolate in your mouth. Pretend it's the first time you have ever tasted chocolate. Focus on how this makes you feel. Pay absolute attention to what is happening in your mouth. After one or two minutes, you can swallow the chocolate.

How does this experience compare to how you normally eat chocolate? Does it taste better than usual? Sometimes you eat without really noticing it, you may taste the first bite but the rest is on autopilot. This mindfulness exercise is closely tied to gratitude because of the conscious softening of your perspective on the mundane day-to-day routines. It enhances your joy by focusing on the smaller things in life. If you like this exercise, try eating a whole meal with conscious attention.

The inner smile: Think of something that makes you smile – it could be a really funny scene from a TV show or the face of a child or someone else you love. Allow yourself to physically smile and as you go deeper into the feeling of happiness and joy, start to feel your heart open up and expand. Begin to relax into the state of pure joy and love. If your mind drifts off, gently bring it back to the image and reconnect to the feelings of joy, happiness and love. Let the energy of this emotion flow all around you and just stay in this space. Try this for a minimum of five minutes and then build up to fifteen.

After practice you will be able to summon up this exercise anywhere at any time – a great tool for battling office politics.

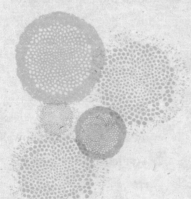

STEP 12

Embracing a New
Version of Life

If you are reading this chapter, then you have possibly made the decision to stop trying for a 'traditional' family. It may feel like the fertility roller-coaster is still racing down the tracks with emotions flying everywhere, or perhaps it has come to an abrupt stop, leaving you with dishevelled hair and white knuckles. Be patient with yourself and your partner as you begin to reconnect to solid ground. Life has altered since you began this ride. With the old dream now receding, you'll begin to find space on your life canvas opening up.

Spending time designing and orchestrating a meaningful and fulfilling life is not about denying the pain and grief of lost parenthood. The black box will be on the canvas too, but it's what also fills the space that will determine how well your new and unexpected life treats you. You are finally back in the driver's seat, and as much as this is not what you wanted or expected, it doesn't mean the future has to be sad, bad or even second rate. There are many inspirational women in the world who live richly rewarding lives without kids: Helen Mirren, Ellen DeGeneres or Cameron Diaz, for example – and that's without looking at your own local networks. I once coached a woman who, at forty-two, had actively chosen not to have children and repeatedly met resistance and social stigma in the workforce. Despite a significant rise in the number of childfree households since the 1950s and the social commentary to match, there is still ground-level resistance, covertly disguised behind supposedly innocent enquiries like 'So why don't you have any kids?'

Few people would look at a childless man and question why he doesn't have kids, but somehow it's been hardwired into our collective unconscious that women should. Try not to take it personally – you are a pioneer in this mode of living. It may not be common, but it's certainly not wrong. It is your generation's responsibility to lay down the new social fabric of acceptability for future generations. Bet you didn't think your Plan B would leave such a legacy, did you?

So, what next? Those three little words can sometimes seem more challenging than the first trip to the moon. Firstly, you need to discover your destination. I would suggest setting a broad intention around living a happy, meaningful and fulfilling life. You don't need to know exactly what that looks like right now, but setting the intention is strong enough to plant the seeds. Once you make the decision to own this reality, your brain will switch gears and seek out the tools and resources needed to make it happen.

Breaking down this intention into lifestyle bites means understanding, personalising and executing the formulas for happiness, meaning and fulfilment. Let's start with happiness.

The American psychologist Dr Martin Seligman, in his book *Authentic Happiness*, details the formula for happiness as $H=S+C+V$, where (H) is happiness; (S) is the genetic set point for happiness; (C) is your circumstances and (V) is factors under your control. We each have a set point of happiness, which normally recalibrates after a major life event. For example, winning the lottery or becoming paraplegic would cause major spikes in happiness and unhappiness levels but these would eventually return close to previously experienced levels of happiness. This could be good information to hang onto. Even though life is never as expected, your happiness levels will hopefully restore to your pre-fertility issue levels. The factors under your control are the most important aspect here. These factors are your line of direct responsibility on how to invest in your happiness. Daily exercises to access the flow of happiness are a simple and yet profound way of making the difference. Tools and exercises such as gratitude lists, random acts of kindness, and learning how to still your mind all assist to prolong states of happiness that otherwise tend to be fleeting. There is no magic pill or epiphany waiting to unlock the secret door to unlimited happiness – it's choosing to integrate happiness tools into your day that makes the difference.

Authentic life purpose

Authenticity is the ability to not only know yourself, but to live your life according to your truth. A sense of meaning can stem from knowing what's important to you. If you are not sure what gives your life meaning, then try writing an obituary for yourself. As morbid as it sounds, it's a great way to look at your life and recall the qualities and accomplishments that have been part of your life to date. Seeing how you've spent your time so far will provide insight into what brought you the most enjoyment and satisfaction, as well as the impact you've made on people and projects. You may uncover a pattern where your core values are expressed or that specific needs repeatedly appeared either fulfilled or unfulfilled.

Coaching Exercise: Pinpoint Your Values

The following exercise is one I often use with clients to explore their values. Take a piece of paper and list all the possible values that resonate with you. Write down as many needs and values as possible – they can be values you live by or wish to have more of. Once your list is complete, pick out the most relevant to you and break them down into groups, summarising each group with one word that best represents the group value.

Here is a list of possible values to get your creative juices flowing:

Adventure	Happiness	Positivity
Ambition	Harmony	Power
Animals	Health	Quietness
Art	Humour	Relationships
Authenticity	Inspiring others	Respect
Balance	Intelligence	Risks
Community	Justice	Security
Compassion	Kindness	Spirituality
Creativity	Knowledge	Style
Environment	Leadership	Support
Expertise	Love	Tidiness
Family	Making a	Time
Fashion	difference	Tolerance
Financial security	Nature	Trust
Friendship	Passion	Understanding
Fun	Personal growth	

After grouping and defining your values, you should be left with a list of about three to six values. Go through each area of your life, such as relationship, work, family, home and general wellbeing, and see where each value is currently being fulfilled. For example, a client whose value is adventure but works in an office and has no hobbies would not be living authentically to that value. Defining what adventure means to them and then committing to the relevant adventurous activities would help bring that value into their life. I have found when people live authentically to their values they often find their tribe and consequently build social networks that feed and nurture their soul.

It's not always appropriate to have each value expressed in each area of your life, but seek out the opportunities to bring you and your values into greater alignment. You can also stick each value on your vision board to remind you where to place your focus.

Defining our needs

Needs are very similar to values — you can't live an authentically meaningful life if you refuse to ask for what you need. So many of us grow up with the notion it is better to let yourself down than to disappoint other people. Of course it is a great human quality to put the wellbeing of your family, friends and colleagues high on your priority list, but not to your own detriment. Remember that instruction on a plane — place your oxygen mask on first before you assist anyone else? It's impossible to serve others properly if your energy tank is depleted.

Perhaps you feel that the risk of upsetting someone is more important than your own wellbeing? Maybe it is easier to wear your own disappointment than let a friend down?

Getting really clear on what exactly it is you need and then asking for it is a huge step toward self-empowerment and living a fulfilling life.

Similar to the values exercise, list all of the things you need in your life to function. These may include feeling appreciated, alone time, a sense of belonging, being respected, sharing household chores, drinking great coffee or exercising. When your needs are met you feel uplifted, energised or possibly relaxed and grounded – most importantly, you are not left wanting or feeling deprived. If there is an area of your life that persistently feels unsettled or occasionally causes aggravation, you may find an unfulfilled need seeking attention. It's hard to enjoy life when you aren't getting your needs met.

Miriam and her partner had 'six children', as she liked to call them – one horse, two dogs, two cats, one bird. After redefining the word 'family' to include their four-legged and feathered friends, she felt complete and safe knowing life would not include a biological baby of their own – their pets were deeply loved and brought much happiness and fulfilment. Miriam learned to own her values of love and compassion, and shifted her focus away from 'destination: baby' and onto the family she was already living with. Her partner also moved into this space of thinking and gradually Miriam began to own her needs to share the responsibility of their alternative babies.

Learning how to design your life to express your values, honour your needs and fully savour the pleasures of life will automatically elevate your state of happiness and fulfilment. But research shows people intrinsically need more for a deeply meaningful life. Looking outside the self and finding purpose in your contribution to a cause greater and longer lasting than you is also key to living a purposeful and fulfilling life – not to mention the benefits to your physical and emotional wellbeing.

Discovering what gives your life meaning may take time. Only you know. Perhaps you are a member of a religion, charity, society or invested in the wellbeing of others in some other way? You may already have established ties to an organisation years ago but let your commitment slip. Revisit where your interests lie. Maybe you have become passionate about a new cause since beginning your fertility journey? Notice where your emotions get fired up; you may feel a sense of injustice or an inner calling. Get clear on where, how and what you could contribute of your time, energy and resources, and begin to take the steps needed to deepen the sense of meaning in your life. This does not mean you walk away from the pleasurable activities that bring joy – no one is asking you to be a saint. Interestingly, by engaging in the activities that bring you greater joy and happiness, you will in turn have more positive energy to contribute to causes greater than yourself, which in turn contribute to your overall happiness.

Engaging fulfilment

The next criterion in the equation is engagement – the key to a sense of fulfilment. Work is an obvious place to secure fulfilment. We spend a huge proportion of our lives at work so it's important to do something for more reasons than just paying the bills. Feeling engaged in work is likened to the term 'being in the flow'. This is when we lose track of time and immerse ourselves in the activity, moment to moment. Your attention is so absorbed in the present, you're unaware of any distractions both inside and outside your head. Being in the flow can occur when playing a musical instrument, skiing down the most perfect slope, on the sports field, delivering a keynote speech or even baking a special cake. Engaging in work that offers you the opportunity to get in the flow may provide you with an undiscovered wealth of satisfaction you didn't even know possible. Be totally honest with yourself and rank your job on a scale of 1 to 10 for its fulfilment. Are you happy with your score? If your intention is to live a happy, meaningful and purposeful life, this means spending your days how you wish to spend your life, doing something you can engage in. You are worthy of a rewarding career.

Of course, finding your flow at work may not be possible right now, so try integrating some non-work activities into your life. List all the hobbies, holidays, sports or events you enjoy and schedule them into the year. Many of my clients have joined evening walking groups that take them on weekly walks as well as treks across the globe. This activity has rolled exercise, adventure and new friendships all in one. In other words, go with the flow and then reap what you sow.

Your fertility journey may have taken you away from some of the relationships you once enjoyed or perhaps it has provided you with new friendships. Either way, feeling fully engaged in your relationships allows the energy of belonging and possibility to flow. Being present to the people in your life and truly honouring the time you have together can bring tremendous joy and satisfaction. You often play many roles in your life without even realising they exist. Most roles involve being a daughter, wife, sister, aunty, godmother, friend, mentor, work colleague, boss, neighbour, student or something like that. How often do you feel truly engaged in your own roles? Are there some areas you would like to improve? Or maybe pull back from?

Witnessing how you act with certain people is useful to distinguish who is going to be part of this new chapter in your life. It's down to you to enrich your life with the people who add value and beauty. As this new time unfolds you may even choose to seek out like-minded souls to share interests and experiences with. Of course, your partner needs to be number one on your list. Few relationships survive the perils of fertility struggles unscathed. Now is the time to deepen your connection and determine who you wish to be as a couple. A relationship isn't a real relationship before it has been challenged.

It's down to you

I hope by now the idea that what you focus on becomes your reality has really sunk in. You do not have the luxury of harbouring shabby, lazy and sabotaging thoughts — they are a dangerous threat to your wellbeing. Taking ownership of this new and unexpected life path is only down to one person — you. As daunting as it may feel, you will thank yourself in the long run for investing in your happiness. You may already carry a suitcase of regrets, but adding to them will not change anything or improve your circumstances. Make the decision to find new purpose in your life. Cover your vision board in images that represent this next chapter. Try writing a mission statement to encompass your vision, values and purpose. It can be as long as you want, but ideally a short paragraph will help keep you grounded as you navigate through your days.

A mission statement is traditionally used in business to guide the decision-making process and keep it accountable to the company's goals and vision. Used personally, it is an anchor to help articulate your purpose on the planet. You may already know your calling or perhaps you have never really considered it before. Creating a mission statement helps quiet the mind chatter and clearly distinguishes between what decisions and circumstances take you toward your life purpose and what takes you away. Here is an example of the mission statement of a past client who was a financial planner:

> I choose to live each day working toward my vision
> of contented happiness and commit to daily steps
> to nurture myself, my partner and our life. I am fully
> engaged at work and make an active contribution to
> the improvement of my clients' wealth. I use my skills as
> an open communicator to inspire and motivate people
> to take responsibility of their finances. My life is a living
> expression of my values of love and respect, and in
> doing so I feel happiness and satisfaction.

To remind you again, your Plan B does not have to be second rate – it's not what you wanted, but in time you may come to love the new life you have created. Keep an open heart and listen to your inner voice, which is always there waiting to offer guidance as you return to the world. Designing the new and empowered version of you is something to be extremely proud of. Not every woman could stand in your shoes and endure the fertility roller-coaster, least of all walk away from it with the determination and plan to live a meaningful and fulfilling life with or without children.

Never, never, never forget your importance. You have so much to offer the world exactly as you are.

Coaching Exercise: Write Your Future

On page 146 is a Life Balance Chart, which will help analyse your level of satisfaction and balance in your life. Each section represents an area of your life, but feel free to change or add new titles if there are additional areas in your life.

Using a scale of 1 (very unsatisfied) to 10 (very satisfied), begin to think about each specific aspect of your life. I have included some questions below to get you thinking.

Score each area of your life based on how you feel right now. Join the numbers with a line to create your personal shape. This represents how you feel today about your life.

Life Balance Chart Questions:

Me

- Do I treat myself as I would my best friend?
- How much do I love/like myself?
- Do I respect myself?
- How authentic am I?

Partner

- How clear are the expectations and roles in our relationship?
- How committed am I to my relationship?
- Are my needs being met by my partner?

Home environment

- How much do I like my neighbourhood?
- Does my home nurture me?
- Am I happy with my home?

Health and wellbeing

- Do I exercise and have a healthy diet?
- How comfortable am I with my state of mind?
- Do I have a positive self-image?

Rest and relaxation

- How effectively do I deal with stress?
- Do I give myself permission to be offline and rest my mind?
- How much time do I spend in my creative zone?
- Am I comfortable saying no to others and yes to myself?

Social life

- How do I feel about the quality of friendships I have?
- Am I satisfied with my level of social activities?
- Do I have room for improvement with my social life?

Career/business

- Do I enjoy what I do for work?
- How clear is my future career/business development?
- Am I happy with my income?
- Is my work environment – for example, company values, colleagues – in alignment with who I am?

Family

- What is the state of my relationship with my parents?
- How do I feel about my relationship with my siblings?
- Are there any family feuds that have an impact on my relationships?

Finances

- Do I feel empowered or petrified by my finances?
- How often do I give adequate time to organising finances?
- Am I clear on my path to financial freedom?
- Do I have more positive or negative thoughts around money?

Spirituality

- Am I clear about my religious or spiritual beliefs?
- How connected do I feel to the rest of the world?
- Do I practise the power of prayer or meditation?
- How peaceful do I feel in my life?

The areas where you scored low are now opportunities to improve your life. Using the MAP your MOVE exercise on page 107, you can set yourself specific goals relating to each area.

Try using a monthly timeframe in the early days of your post-fertility journey. Then move to quarterly goals. Lots of small wins and ticks on the to-do list are much more motivating and far better for the soul than grandiose, unachievable goals.

The Life Balance Chart

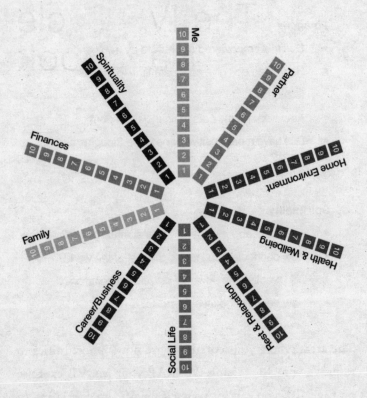

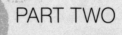

PART TWO

The IVF Cycle
Handbook

The IVF Experience

by Dr Devora Lieberman

Every month in a natural cycle, depending on her age, a woman will have anywhere from one to thirty small follicles begin to grow from the start of her period. Follicles are little fluid-filled cysts that contain immature eggs. With the follicle stimulating hormone (FSH) that her pituitary gland produces, only one of those follicles will grow, dominate and subsequently ovulate. The rest will be reabsorbed by the ovary, never to be used again.

With in vitro fertilisation (IVF) we take advantage of all of those follicles and, through injections of FSH, encourage ideally half-a-dozen to a dozen follicles to mature. The eggs are collected transvaginally under ultrasound guidance and are then mixed with sperm to enable fertilisation. The resulting embryos are cultured for several days and then one (or sometimes two) embryos are transferred back to the uterus. Ideally, there will be more embryos that can be frozen for later use.

Media reports of IVF treatment make the process seem pretty horrific – drugs that make you feel and behave worse than the most severe PMT imaginable, huge needles that are painfully injected into the buttocks, along with endless ultrasounds and blood tests, which consume all of a woman's waking hours.

The good news is that IVF treatments have become much more woman-friendly in the past ten years. There are newer treatment protocols that, for many, require fewer injections and hormonal ups and downs. The injections are now given via pen-like devices with tiny needles, and are no worse than the smallest GP jab. Most clinics will do their very best to work with a woman's busy life; they open early so a woman can have her blood tests and ultrasounds and then get on with her day. I'd estimate that more than ninety-five per cent of my patients say to me at the end of a cycle, 'Gee, Devora, that wasn't nearly as bad as I expected.' Of course, their expectations were probably quite low to begin with.

People often talk about the emotional roller-coaster of IVF. I'd suggest that all my patients trying to conceive have been on an emotional roller-coaster long before they started IVF: taking their basal body temperature every morning, peeing on sticks to try to determine if they're ovulating or not, having acupuncture, swallowing natural and herbal remedies, eating pineapple core – you name it,

I've probably heard of it. The roller-coaster ride may be exaggerated, but many people tell me that when they get to IVF they have a newfound sense of control, and with that thought in mind, I hope this handbook helps you to navigate the highs and the lows of treatment.

Claire has designed a series of things to consider and tasks for each of the stages of IVF treatment, from the first injection through to the dreaded two-week wait. Of course, every woman will experience an IVF cycle in her own unique way, but there are certainly some common themes that I see among my patients. Some women tell me that they are excited about starting treatment, after floundering in the dark for so long, relying on ovulation predictor kits and internet forums for support. Others find it overwhelming and frightening. Often it's a fear of the unknown, or a very real needle phobia.

You are not the first person to experience these emotions, and it probably wouldn't be normal if you weren't just a little bit apprehensive, either. When going through treatment, you should have an entire team of people all devoted to doing everything possible to support you and achieve your very best outcome. It's important that you feel that you can get that support from your clinical team – your doctor, nurses, scientists, counsellors – they are all there to help.

But I think the greatest fear for the women and couples I see is a fear of failure. There are so many hurdles to be tackled: ovaries must respond to stimulation, mature eggs must be collected that can then fertilise normally, then there is the gauntlet of embryo development, and, of course, the pregnancy test. For many women, it doesn't stop there, especially if there is a history of miscarriage.

This handbook is designed to help you at every stage. No matter what the outcome of your fertility treatment, we hope that this process will help you increase your resilience and become the very best you that you can be.

How to use this handbook

The first half of this book takes a big-picture approach to tackling some of the issues surrounding an experience of infertility. This second half, the handbook, is designed to give you practical information, things to consider and tasks to increase your wellbeing through each stage of the IVF cycle.

The number one thing to remember is to remain true to your journal – I hope it is proving a helpful ally on this journey. Keep writing insights and answers to the questions in each section below. This handbook is ideally used as a base for you to jump backward and forward to seek out the best advice and tools suited to your needs at any specific time. There is no set course, just use your intuition as you need. Sometimes it's good to flick open the whole book and read whatever jumps out at you. I have learned many life lessons from various books this way, especially when I am time poor and in need of some instant inspiration.

You may not be following the exact IVF path as listed here, and that's okay. All countries, clinics and specialists use their own techniques, but you will find a core theme you can relate to.

Please remember to meet yourself exactly where you are, give yourself permission to feel what you need to feel, accept what is and what isn't, and most of all, be kind and compassionate to the beautiful woman you are.

MILESTONE 1

The Injection Phase

There are several different ways that your ovaries can be stimulated, depending on your individual circumstances and the requirements of your clinic. Some women will take an oral contraceptive for a few weeks to 'time' their cycle; others will start with their regular period. There is no one best stimulation protocol, and if you have questions or concerns about what is right for you, you should discuss these with your doctor.

Dr Devora Lieberman

Finally it's here, no more waiting for the cycle to begin. You have done the research, listened to the advice and embraced the possibility of starting a family. You may feel anything from excited and nervous to ambivalent. All feelings are okay; remember not to judge them or give them too much importance as they can distract you from the tasks at hand.

This first week may leave you feeling like you have landed in the front seat of a roller-coaster. In a short space of time, not only will you be facing new physical challenges, but emotionally, things may seem overwhelming and stressful too. It is important to remain calm and focused by setting realistic expectations for yourself, your partner and the process itself.

Things to consider
Conquering daily injections

The act of daily self-injecting may provoke anxiety and stress, especially if you are uncomfortable with needles. As you endure this necessary but unpleasant task, it will help to remind yourself of the big picture and the reasons you are doing this. Remember to ask for help if you need it. Injections may be out of your comfort zone at first, but with practice they can soon become easy. Many women even feel empowered as they overcome their fear of needles. Think of something else that you have felt uncomfortable about, but that became straightforward and easy once you mastered.

MY TASKS:

What is my positive focus point?

When else have I mastered a challenging activity?

Get organised

Trying to fit another commitment into your busy life may be a squeeze, so setting up an efficient system to manage your time will overcome a lot of the stress and anxiety. Sit down with a pen and paper and plan your activities from Monday to Sunday. Allocate a block of time in your diary to prepare and submit any paperwork required. The timing and practicalities of injections needs to be well thought out and organised in advance, so integrate the injection times into your diary so you know exactly where you and your partner will be.

MY TASKS:

On a scale of 1–10, how organised do I feel right now?

What steps do I need to take to get more organised?

Do I need any apps, diaries or calendars to help streamline my organisation?

Do I need to temporarily give up anything to free space in my day?

Don't make assumptions, get the facts

While you are going through this fertility process it's only natural many questions will crop up. Your clinic will have all the answers, to the extent that there are any. Human biology can be complicated, and your body, eggs and embryos don't always do what you'd like them to. Keep asking questions until you get an answer that takes you out of stressful uncertainty and assumption, and into a place of confidence, knowing you have the right information. Please refer back to Step 3: Letting Go of Expectations on page 21 for more information about your brain's response to certainty.

> **MY TASKS:**
>
> What do I need to know to feel more empowered on this journey?
>
> How empowered do I feel with my current knowledge?
>
> Does my partner have any unanswered questions?

Needs and wants

One simple and effective style of communicating your needs and wants is to clearly state:

- The situation from a non-objective point of view such as 'There are a lot of demands on my time at the moment.'
- How that makes you feel – 'I'm feeling very stressed as a result.'
- What you need as a solution – 'What I really want is to not feel obligated to attend family functions in April.'
- How that lands with the listener – 'How does that sound to you?'

It can be challenging to express your needs from an assertive place but the consequences of not doing so can be far more damaging. Step 8: Handling Family and Friends on page 87 offers additional information on communication.

> **MY TASKS:**
>
> What do I need and want right now from my partner and my family and friends?
>
> What is it costing me to not have this?
>
> When will I sit down and discuss this with the people who are important to me?

This may be your second or more cycle. It is important to use the experience of your previous cycles to your advantage. Spend a moment recalling any past IVF journeys and what you learned from those experiences. How will this make you stronger this time around? Do you wish to do something differently this time? How can you build on what you learned about yourself, your partner and the process from the previous cycles so you are better informed and ready for this one? Get prepared: you know what lies ahead, so make sure you have the resources in place to assist your new IVF cycle.

> **MY TASKS:**
>
> How am I approaching this new cycle differently?
>
> What positive advice would I give to my best friend if she were in my shoes?
>
> Do I need to take that advice myself?

The magic of a letting-go balloon

Try sending any negative thoughts away in a letting-go balloon. Sit quietly and recall any grievances that you wish to release. Breathe in each of those past experiences and negative thoughts, then blow them into an imaginary balloon. For example, 'This cycle isn't going to work', or 'I can't stand the stress of all these injections'. When the balloon is fully blown up, tie an imaginary knot and let it float away into the distance, taking with it all the stress those thoughts were causing you. This is a great tool to use before you go to sleep at night, or if you are one of those people who wake up in the early hours with a head full of worries.

MY TASK:

Write a list of all those niggling grievances that distract you and weigh heavily on your mind. Now consider:

- What are some of the impacts playing out in my life because of these grievances?
- If I am really honest with myself, does it serve me to hang on to them? Do I need to be 'right' or is there a more peaceful path?

MILESTONE 2

The Egg Collection

Egg collection involves the aspiration of the fluid from the follicles that will, hopefully, contain eggs. The procedure is carried out through the vagina on each side of the cervix, and is guided by transvaginal ultrasound. In most IVF clinics, this is done under sedation or even a general anaesthetic, but local anaesthetic with pain relief is also an option.

Dr Devora Lieberman

You have successfully navigated your way through the self-injection phase. Well done! Now it's time to take stock and gather your resources to smoothly transition through the next stage, which is egg collection. New and old challenges may lie ahead. Some women experience stress trying to cram the numerous scans and blood tests into an already tight daily schedule. Others may focus on the weight of the unknown or heightened anxiety and stress after obtaining poor past results. No matter what feelings or concerns you are experiencing, remember they are all valid and important to address. Think of them as little gifts of enlightenment, as challenging as that may be. The conscious act of choosing to use this experience as a catalyst to empower you will enable you to create a toolkit of resilience and positivity to carry with you through life.

Things to consider
Dealing with uncertainty

This next week may present an array of uncertainty regarding trigger injections, follicle development, day surgery or embryo development. A quick recap of Step 3: Letting Go of Expectations on page 21 will remind you of the brain mechanics behind the emotive power of uncertainty.

MY TASKS:

What do I need to know to feel comfortable and
    empowered?

On a scale of 1 to 10, how well do I handle uncertainty?
    How do I tend to react to it?

What do I need to learn about myself to become more
    comfortable with uncertainty?

Comfort zone

Life is a series of comfort zone expansions: each time you become comfortable with a new challenge or a new situation, it becomes part of your comfort zone. So however challenged you feel at the moment with what you have to do, stick with it, and your comfort zone will catch up. Try to leave any past bad experiences or negativity from previous cycles in the old comfort zone so they don't taint your experience when embracing a new one. Step 5: A Conversation with Fear on page 45 offers more information on dealing with this milestone.

> **MY TASKS:**
>
> What have I done in the past that has truly challenged me to my core?
>
> What did I learn about myself as a result of committing to overcoming that?
>
> What strengths do I possess that can help me now?

Nurture and balance

Investing in your emotional wellbeing and integrating self-nurturing activities into your week is essential right now. Refer back to Step 7: Building Your Emotional Toolkit on page 75 and refresh your memory. Self-care may slip to the bottom of the priority list, but without it you are making the journey unnecessarily hard. Consciously balancing a stressful activity with a nurturing one is enough to help keep the balance and, therefore, motivation.

> **MY TASKS:**
>
> What are my top ten favourite ways to pamper myself?
>
> Why is it important for me to balance this IVF with self-nurturing?
>
> How am I going to ensure I commit to my wellbeing?

Staying positive on those hard days

Sometimes it can get really hard to stay motivated and positive – especially when there have been disappointments and setbacks and you feel you are getting nowhere. On those types of days, when you just don't seem to be able to get your act together, try a visualisation to help you focus on the present and get into motion.

Go forward in your mind to the end of the day and look back. Imagine how you will feel if you have spent the day feeling sorry for yourself, procrastinating and not really achieving anything you know you need to do.

Now imagine how you will feel if you have put your negative feelings aside and just got on with some of the things you know you have – and indeed want – to do, be they part of the fertility process or other tasks.

Now ask yourself: 'What can I do now to make me feel good at the end of this day?'

> **MY TASKS:**
>
> What can I do to help myself recognise one of those
> hard days and break its spell?
>
> If I'm having a hard day, what can I say to myself that
> is loving, kind and compassionate to help me get
> through?

Being a team

The harmony of your relationship with your partner and
keeping connected to them is vital at this important time.
Keep the communication paths between you open, be they
written, verbal or physical. Use active listening so you really
understand what the other person is saying – relay back to
them what they have told you they are feeling, not just what
you think they feel. Rather than challenging or disagreeing
with them, establish the rule that each person's reality of the
situation is valid and there are no universals truths or right
and wrongs – you are a team working toward the same goal.
Confronting and accepting your emotions together can help
you move beyond them so they don't cause stress. Step 9:
Relationship Bumps on page 95 offers more tips on this.

> **MY TASKS:**
>
> How well do I express myself to my partner? Do they
> complain they don't understand where I'm coming
> from, or I of them?

What are my natural defence mechanisms when
  under stress? Do they serve the harmony of my
  relationship?
How can we ensure we remain connected even during
  stressful times?

Embryo Transfer

The transfer of the embryo to the uterus is straightforward, almost like having a pap smear. A speculum is placed in the vagina and a fine plastic catheter that has been loaded with the embryo is passed through the cervix into the uterus.

Dr Devora Lieberman

Having negotiated and accomplished the challenges of the past few weeks, you and your partner deserve to congratulate each other on completing the journey so far.

Life now takes on a different pace as the demands on your time begin to slow down. Once the embryo transfer is complete, the wait begins. Women frequently express the heightened stress and anxiety around managing this phase.

As you start to reclaim your time it is important to remain focused on the positive and not pander to every doubt and uncertainty that enters your mind.

Things to consider
Sharing your wins

Step 3's coaching exercise, 'Cultivate Gratitude' (on page 30), focuses on the retraining of your brain to seek out the positive in a situation. A similar daily empowering and stabilising thing to do with your partner is to share and acknowledge your wins – what has gone well. You may think it has been a dog of a day with no wins, but there will always be something that has worked and deserves acknowledgement.

MY TASKS:

What are three wins I experienced today?

What persistent complaint do I have that could be reframed into a win? For example, 'It's great to have an electricity bill because I have the money to pay for it,' rather than thinking, 'Oh no, not another bill.'

How powerful is the positive part of my brain compared to my crazy monkey negative part? Do I need to address that balance?

Get out of yourself

Sometimes you just need to take time out. Not only physical time out, like going for a walk, but mental time out. Time to fill your mind with something other than the outcome of your fertility process.

Going to a show or taking in a movie, or even reading a good book, can be a really useful way of getting out of your worrisome environment – turning off and tuning out. And that in itself can be re-energising because it fills your mind with something else to think about. Of course, you need to pick your show, movie or book carefully, like a lively musical, a good thriller, or historical romance; choose something that will engage your thoughts and take them away from your anxieties. Think of this time out as being similar to turning your computer completely off rather than just leaving it in sleep mode, which still burns up energy.

MY TASKS:

If I were to give myself permission to get out of my IVF
    thoughts, what would I want to do?
How can I make that happen this week?
Do I need to bring anyone else in on this to make it more
    achievable?

Clearing the air

As Step 9: Relationship Bumps on page 95 emphasises, your relationship needs to be supportive at this time. Using the phrase 'What do I feel like saying?' is a great way to get things out of your system and clear up any little annoyances or festering misunderstandings so you can both go forward without resentments or unintentional arguments draining your energy.

MY TASKS:

Do I need to clear the air about anything in particular?

What routine do my partner and I need to establish in
order to ensure we keep our relationship space
clear and clean?

Banishing negativity

Focusing on the positives in your life is one vital key to reducing additional stress and unhappiness. Resolve to catch yourself having negative thoughts or saying words such as 'if only' or 'I should have' or dwelling on what you don't have. See Step 2's coaching exercise, 'Learning to Accept' on page 19 to help change your thinking.

MY TASKS:

What are the three things I am most grateful for right now?

What are my Achilles' heels? What do I often hear myself
saying or thinking?

Keeping busy

It is important to fill your waiting time with activities that are going to keep your mind busy and away from the worry and uncertainty of the embryo transfer. It won't be easy to not think about it; it's far too important for that. However, unnecessary worry will not serve you and will not change anything. Below you will find a list of activities that could help distract and empower you at this time.

Exercise is a great stress release. Yoga, walking, dancing, cycling, tai chi, martial arts, Pilates and swimming work wonders. Treat yourself to a massage, pedicure, manicure, facial, concert, watch a favourite movie or read a novel. And if you have any doubts about what you should or shouldn't be doing, ask your clinic. Don't forget to use your emotional toolkit for inspiration.

MY TASKS:

What are my top four favourite things to do?

How will I feel after I have spent some time enjoying each
activity?

Is there any exercise/class/hobby that I have always
wanted to try? Is now the time to start?

Calming the mind

Affirmations are a great way to create a positive mindset as described in the 'Positive Affirmations' exercise in Step 7 on page 82. Repeating a positive sentence either out loud or in your head can help combat sabotaging negative thoughts. Refer back to the list described in the exercise and create some more of your own. Repeat one or more sentences ten times every morning and throughout your day to calm your mind. The coaching exercise 'Getting Through Grief with Mindfulness' on page 123 from Step 11: When Enough is Enough, will also help at this time.

Following is another meditation to achieve calmness and tranquility:

Remember to turn off the phone and sit comfortably on the floor or a chair. Take five slow deep breaths, relaxing the body on each exhale. Begin to witness your thoughts and, without judgement, allow each thought to drift away. Repeat the following as you take deep breaths (you may want to record the affirmation in your own voice to play as you meditate):

- Breathe in light, breathe out fear
- Breathe in hope, breathe out fear
- Breathe in peace, breathe out fear
- Breathe in calmness, breathe out fear
- Breathe in confidence, breathe out fear
- Breathe in trust, breathe out fear

- Breathe in love, breathe out fear
- Breathe in acceptance, breathe out fear.

Then take a moment to harness the tranquility and stillness you create and carry that with you throughout your day, knowing you are only a breath away from inner calm.

MY TASKS:

How important is mental poise and relaxation to me?

What benefits will I get if I commit to focusing my mind on affirmations or a meditation?

Is there a local group I can join to learn more about meditation?

MILESTONE 4

The Waiting Game

You are almost at the finishing line but after such tumultuous events you now have to simply wait for the outcome. The embryo's destiny has been determined. It is either chromosomally normal, or it's not. It has enough energy to keep developing, or it doesn't. It will take around two weeks before you know whether you have had IVF success or not. There isn't anything you can do to influence the fate of your embryo, for better or worse.

Dr Devora Lieberman

Some couples report a feeling of being sent off into the wilderness during the two-week wait, which is in stark contrast to the previous support they had from their clinic. However, you are not really alone. This is merely the next phase of your journey, as you may remember from previous cycles, and this downtime is the perfect opportunity to get yourself emotionally ready for the pregnancy test to come.

Things to consider
Future thinking

Of course you know there are no guarantees on the results of your fertility program, so it's natural to find it stressful to be so out of control, and to only be able to hope and pray for the outcome you want. But what you do have control over is what you will do when the cycle is finished – whatever the result.

Now could be the time to plan for a short break or holiday with your partner, away from the burden of the last few weeks. Choose a relaxing and nurturing environment where you can reconnect.

MY TASKS:

What sort of nurturing do I need to commit to in order to
    bring us back to a balance post cycle?
What am I going to do about this or when am I going to
    book something?

Seek first to understand and then be understood

This phrase comes from Stephen R. Covey, who wrote *The 7 Habits of Highly Effective People*, and it's about trying to understand negative words and behaviours rather than reacting to them. Look below the surface of particular comments or actions you may see as unwarranted negativity and try to understand what is behind the words. By being willing to compassionately ask and discover what is really going on, you reduce the chance of misunderstandings and conflict. As you may have already discovered, the fertility process is often not a solo act and it can affect those around you almost as much as it affects you. Understand those effects and life will be easier and less stressful for all.

MY TASKS:

What sort of statements are really getting under my skin of late?

Do I need to understand someone with more compassion than I am currently granting them?

How does my opinion of certain people or behaviours cause me stress? How can I view this with more calm?

Tolerances

Now could be the ideal time to look around you and address and handle all those little things you are just tolerating or putting up with in your life – things you may not even realise are causing you stress, but once handled will make for an easier and more peaceful journey. Look around your home, your office, your car, your kitchen, your wardrobe. Are there appliances that need repairing so that every time you go to use them you won't get annoyed or frustrated? As you go through the day, make a note of those things you are just putting up with and resolve to handle at least one of them each week.

MY TASKS:

What are all of those tolerations that cause little bubbles of stress throughout my day?

What do I choose to do with them?

How can the decisions I make now improve my life, moving forward?

Make the most of your time

With so many waiting days ahead, you and your partner may feel the emotional ups and downs intensify as you have more time on your hands. By shifting your perception you can reframe this wait into an opportunity for cementing your emotional toolkit. This is valuable time to reflect on your experience so far, both as an individual and as a couple. Invest time writing in your journal to explore and release emotions from your system. A great distraction is decluttering, which is a good way to cleanse the home and also the soul. You will find that as you clear out your physical space, your mental space also becomes clearer. Clearing out the old and allowing new energy into your environment can help create feelings of empowerment and clarity. Maybe start with your wardrobe or some other cluttered space, then move on to sort out something like your photo collection. You could even create an impressive photo album in the process!

> **MY TASKS:**
>
> Where do I have clutter in my life?
>
> What do I need to do in order to create room in my life to sort this out once and for all?
>
> What are the top three decluttering activities I can commit to that will bring the greatest feeling of satisfaction?

Making plans

Your previous experience may be hindering your ability to think clearly. If this isn't your first cycle, remember that this one is completely different from those that came before it. Find some quiet time in the days ahead to sit down and visualise the actual pregnancy test experience from both a positive and negative result perspective. See it as a movie playing in your mind's eye. Notice any feelings or thoughts that arise. When you feel you have gathered all the information you can from the scene, write down how you envisioned the best possible outcome for each result. You may not be able to control the results, but you can control your response. By taking charge and mentally visiting each scenario, you become responsible for ensuring you are as prepared as possible to proactively and positively deal with the outcome.

You can use this exercise to prepare for any aspect of your treatment. Remember, you have the power to confront each challenge with the strength and determination this journey has brought out of you so far.

> **MY TASKS:**
>
> As confronting as this may be, what benefit will I have by visiting each possible scenario?
>
> When do I have the time to fully engage in this exercise and allow myself to feel with no judgement?
>
> How can I use what I learn from this exercise to become more empowered when I take the test?

Family and friends' support

You may already know how you wish to manage your friends' and family's support based on a previous experience and from the advice shared in Step 8: Handling Family and Friends on page 87. However, it's always refreshing to review exactly where you stand. Friends and family can be both a blessing and a hindrance at this very challenging time. As much as you need the understanding and compassion of your loved ones, it can be hard to clearly express what is happening to you when your thoughts and feelings are so raw and scattered in your own head. Some people may not truly understand the process or be sensitive to how you may be feeling. Others will be a rock of support and contribute much to the success of your experience.

It is important to know where to go for real emotional support. Start by separating your family and friends into lists under the headings 'Energising' or 'Energy Zapping'. The names on your energising list are your support team, the people you can count on confidently to make you feel better rather than drag you down. Next you will need to run through the pros and cons of when and how to communicate with those on your support team. These people will want to help but may not know how. Be willing to always explain exactly what you need from them so they feel empowered to help you.

MY TASKS:

What criteria shall I use to judge who is energising and
    who is energy zapping?

Now I know who truly supports me, what can I do with
    this knowledge to help me?

How can I keep my precious energy safe from the
    energy vampires in my life?

MILESTONE 5

Taking the Test

Most clinics will do a blood test looking for pregnancy hormone (hCG) about sixteen days after the egg collection. At that point, the levels should be high enough to give a definitive yes or no. Home pregnancy tests are notoriously unreliable at low levels, so even if you have had a negative home test (which most clinics would discourage using), it is important to get confirmation. Some people may be happily surprised!

Dr Devora Lieberman

Y ou have had the blood test and, hopefully, the dust is starting to settle and you can begin to think about the impact of the results. If you are pregnant, congratulations! You will now be eagerly waiting for the six- to seven-week scan. If you are not pregnant, it is time to reflect and to consider the next path of action toward achieving your goal of parenthood. You might want to look at frozen embryo transfer, if you were fortunate to have embryos stored. You may want to start another IVF cycle straightaway. Or maybe you don't have the financial resources, or otherwise, to keep going? All three paths present new questions and challenges that require the same degree of dedication and courage that this whole journey has demanded of you and your partner.

Pregnant
Embarking on parenthood

Finally the dream becomes a reality. You are pregnant! While you may be feeling joy and excitement, you know to hold your final jubilation until you are given the official green light. However, now is the perfect time to start indulging in the wealth of pregnancy books and online information. Start by allocating a specific folder to store interesting articles, websites or booklets. Not only will each stage of pregnancy require research, such as the type of medical care you select, dietary requirements and exercise recommendations, but you and your partner must now start to think about the type of parents you choose to be. If you haven't already done so, begin to share your parenting beliefs and experiences. Think about and discuss what type of parents you want to be. Don't just do something because it was how you were brought up – develop your own parenting strategies. A good way to start is by comparing how you were encouraged and punished as a child and whether, in retrospect, that worked as a parenting strategy. Let it flow from there.

> **MY TASKS:**
>
> What do I most remember from my parents as a child?
>
>> What stands out as good parenting and not-so-good parenting?
>
> How can I positively approach this next stage so I feel empowered throughout?

Acknowledge your courage

It's time to give yourself a pat on the back and acknowledge the courage and commitment it has taken to undertake this fertility process. Getting to this stage is a huge achievement and not something to be overlooked. Just remember how strong you and your partner really are to make this choice and stay on track until you achieved your goal. Stop and allow yourselves to relish in the delights of your hard work. If you can conquer this arduous journey, what other great challenges are you capable of overcoming together?

> **MY TASKS:**
>
> What have I learned about myself as a result of this experience?

> What have I learned about my partner and our
>   relationship?
>
> How can we use these insights to move forward to a
>   deeper connection?

Remember to look after your health

As a pregnant woman it is so important to look after your health. You might have set off at the beginning of your fertility process with all good intentions around looking after yourself. But as the weeks have gone by, stress may have overtaken your resolve, and almost without you realising, healthy eating and exercise have slipped out of your focus.

If this has happened to you, now is a good time to remind yourself it is vital to keep healthy. Commit to making sure that each day you nourish your body, your baby and your spirit by eating well, relaxing and doing some exercise.

Boundaries

You may remember how we talked about the importance of setting boundaries around not letting people upset you with negative comments about you or the fertility process you are going through. Now you are pregnant it is still vital to maintain these boundaries. This can be challenging because you don't want to upset people who may mean well, but at the same time, for your own wellbeing and empowerment, you need to let them know firmly that you do not welcome their comments. You are still in those early stages of pregnancy and finding your feet.

If someone oversteps your boundary, try these statements:

- 'I know you mean well, but your comments/opinions are really not helping me and I would ask you not to express them to me.'
- 'I value our friendship and your opinions, but I hope you will understand this is one subject I really don't choose to have conversations about yet.'

And if all else fails: 'Please, I don't wish/choose to discuss this with you and I'd ask you to respect that for the sake of our relationship/friendship.'

Not pregnant (yet)

This is a good time to have a conversation with your doctor. Sometimes things may be more clear once you have been through a cycle and your doctor will have learned a lot about:

- How your ovaries responded to stimulation.
- How your eggs looked.
- How the eggs fertilised.
- How the embryos developed.

Finding a new path to parenthood

So your treatment is not working out as you had hoped. It is heartbreaking, but try not to give in to despair. Remember your goal and the reasons that drove you to this place. Before you begin to tread a new path, such as another round of IVF, egg or sperm donation or adoption, in your journey toward parenthood, gather all the information available to you so you are fully equipped to make educated and informed decisions. Leave no stone unturned. Write out a list of the questions you need answered in order to make a decision and seek out the experts to answer them. Keep a file of your findings and, when you feel you have enough data, prioritise the key factors around your desire for a child. See which path will give you the most support in alignment with your goal. Once your head is satisfied with the answer, check in with your heart. Your intuition is a wise tool, so don't be afraid to listen to it. See Step 11: When Enough is Enough on page 111 for a reminder on accessing your intuition.

Acknowledge your courage

Time to give yourself a pat on the back and acknowledge the courage and commitment it has taken to undertake this fertility process. In fact, whenever you feel your mood going down, just remember how strong you and your partner really are to make this choice and stay on track as long as you have. This formula for courage might help: Courage = Commitment + Doubt + Action. You and your partner have shown great commitment. Through all the doubts and obstacles you have overcome and are yet to face, you constantly took action, and that means you have courage.

Boundaries

At this delicate time it is still vital to maintain your boundaries. This can be challenging because you don't want to upset people who may mean well, but at the same time, for your own wellbeing and empowerment, you need to firmly let them know that you do not welcome their comments. You and your partner do not need to explain anything to anyone. Some suggestions on how to handle this can be found in Step 8: Handling Family and Friends on page 87.

Remember to look after your health

Your health is the number one priority, so if it's taken a backseat of late it's time to schedule some wellbeing commitments such as eating well, relaxing and exercise.

Next steps

Another cycle?

You may just want to jump straight back on the horse. Another treatment cycle could be exactly what feels right for you. But does your partner agree? Before you commit, make sure you are both in the best possible emotional space to go along this path. You are no longer inexperienced – you've gained confidence and knowledge of the expectations of IVF. With your partner, dedicate some quality thinking time (that means no distractions at all) and write a list of all the pros and cons, doubts and fears of another cycle. It's a good idea to start off doing this separately, so you don't influence each other or just agree for the sake of agreeing. Consider all aspects around finances, mood swings, frozen embryos, friends and family, work commitments and your relationship. Then compare what you have both come up with and talk about any areas where you are not in harmony. After this exercise you will both be in a strong position to make the right decision. See the 'Fact Feeler' exercise on page 115 in Step 11 for more on this.

Not pregnant and stopping

If you have reached the decision to stop IVF, I would encourage you to take on board Step 12: Embracing a New Version of Life on page 129. Here you will find tools to redesign what purposeful living means to you. If you haven't reached the decision to stop just yet, maybe give yourself some time to see how you feel, then maybe visit some of the exercises in Step 11: When Enough is Enough on page 111.

I wish you well on your journey, wherever it takes you, and hope this handbook provides something of a toolkit to help you get there.

Resources

Here is a list of resources we encourage you to explore. They are filled with useful information for your fertility journey and provide a platform for your continued learning as you navigate through life.

Publications

Buckingham, Wendy, *Be Your Own Goals Coach*, Class One Productions, Sydney, 2013

Chapman, Gary D, *The Five Love Languages: The Secret to Love that Lasts*, Moody Press, USA, 2010

Covey, Stephen R., *The Seven Habits of Highly Effective People*, Free Press, New York, 1989

Jeffers, Susan, *Feel The Fear … and Do It Anyway*, The Random House Publishing Group, USA, 1987

Kübler-Ross, Elizabeth, and Kessler, David, *On Grief and Grieving: Finding the Meaning of Grief Through the Five Stages of Loss*, Simon & Schuster Ltd, Great Britain, 2005

Rock, David, *Quiet Leadership: Six Steps to Transforming Performance at Work*, HarperCollins Publishers, New York, 2006

Seligman, Dr Martin, *Authentic Happiness: Using the New Positive Psychology to Realize Your Potential for Lasting Fulfillment*, Free Press, New York, 2002

Seligman, Dr Martin, *Learned Optimism: How to Change Your Mind and Your Life*, Vintage Books, New York, 2006

Schwartz, Dr Jeffery M, and Gladding, Dr Rebecca, *You Are Not Your Brain*, Avery, New York, 2011

Online Resources

AUSTRALIA:

AccessAustralia: Australia's National Infertility Network offers a huge range of resources and support for those experiencing fertility problems – www.access.org.au

Donor Conception Support Group of Australia: Membership is made up of people considering or using donor sperm, eggs or embryos, those who already have children conceived on donor programs, adult donor-conceived people and donors – www.dcsg.org.au

SANDS: A self-help support group run by parents who have experienced the death of a baby through miscarriage, still birth or shortly after birth – www.sands.org.au

Bears of Hope Pregnancy & Infant Loss Support: Provides leading support and exceptional care for families who experience the loss of their baby – www.bearsofhope.org.au

Andrology Australia: Provides resources on male reproductive health disorders and their associations with chronic disease – www.andrologyaustralia.org

NEW ZEALAND:

FertilityNZ: The national network for those seeking support and information on fertility problems – www.fertilitynz.org.nz

SANDS: A self-help support group run by parents who have experienced the death of a baby through miscarriage, still birth or shortly after birth – www.sands.org.nz

UNITED STATES OF AMERICA:

RESOLVE: The National Infertility Association: A non-profit, charitable organisation that works to improve the lives of women and men living with infertility – www.resolve.org

The American Fertility Association (The AFA): An inclusive organisation committed to helping people create their families of choice by providing leading-edge outreach programs and timely educational information – www.theafa.org

The Fertility Network: A site connecting to IVF clinics, infertility specialists, egg donation agencies, and other services – www.fertilitynetwork.com

British Infertility Counselling Association (BICA): The only professional association for infertility counsellors and counselling in the UK – www.bica.net

SANDS: A self-help support group run by parents who have experienced the death of a baby through miscarriage, still birth or shortly after birth – www.uk-sands.org

Donor Conception Network: A supportive network of more than 2000 mainly UK-based families with children conceived with donated sperm, eggs or embryos – www.dcnetwork.org

Inspirational Authors

In my research for this book we came across some amazing female warriors who are paving the way for many childless women to follow. They bravely share their fertility journeys and hold their heads high as they pioneer this new frontier of childfree living. We encourage you to seek their wisdom when the time is right for you.

Day, Jody, *Rocking the Life Unexpected: 12 Weeks to Your Plan B for a Meaningful and Fulfilling Life Without Children* – gateway-women.com

Manterfield, Lisa, *I'm Taking My Eggs and Going Home:*
How One Woman Dared to Say No to Motherhood –
lifewithoutbaby.com

Tsigdinos, Pamela Mahoney, *Silent Sorority:*
A (Barren) Woman gets Busy, Angry, Lost and
Found – www.silentsorority.com

Acknowledgements

This book would not have been possible without the support and love of my beautiful husband, Benjamin. My love and gratitude also to our parents, Harry, Lillian, Fred and Carolyn.

Words cannot express my gratitude to Dr Devora Lieberman for her faith, honesty, enthusiasm and continuous support.

My thanks to Emma Hutchinson and Kylie Mason for their advice and expertise in polishing this manuscript.

To my publisher, Sophie Hamley, and agent, Pippa Masson, for making this dream a reality.

To Karen Howard and Khurshida Ajam for opening the fertility door and to every client who walked through it and trusted me with their journey, I thank you with love and gratitude.

Claire Hall